Laryngeal Electromyography

Second Edition

Laryngeal Electromyography

Second Edition

Robert T. Sataloff, M.D., D. M.A.
Steven Mandel, M.D.
Yolanda Heman-Ackah, M.D.
Ramon Mañon-Espaillat, M.D., M.A.
Mona Abaza, M.D.

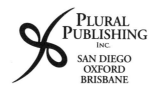

PLURAL
PUBLISHING
INC.
SAN DIEGO
OXFORD
BRISBANE

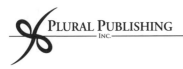

5521 Ruffin Road
San Diego, CA 92123

e-mail: info@pluralpublishing.com
Web site: http://www.pluralpublishing.com

49 Bath Street
Abingdon, Oxfordshire OX14 1EA
United Kingdom

Typeset in 11/13 Garamond by Flanagan's Publishing Services, Inc.
Printed in the United States of America by McNaughton and Gunn

NOTICE TO THE READER

Care has been taken to confirm the accuracy of the indications, procedures, drug
dosages, and diagnosis and remediation protocols presented in this book and to
ensure that they conform to the practices of the general medical and health services communities. However, the authors, editors, and publisher are not responsible for errors or omissions or for any consequences from application of the
information in this book and make no warranty, expressed or implied, with respect
to the currency, completeness, or accuracy of the contents of the publication. The
diagnostic and remediation protocols and the medications described do not necessarily have specific approval by the Food and Drug administration for use in the
disorders and/or diseases and dosages for which they are recommended. Application of this information in a particular situation remains the professional responsibility of the practitioner. Because standards of practice and usage change, it is the
responsibility of the practitioner to keep abreast of revised recommendations,
dosages, and procedures.

ISBN-13: 978-1-59756-005-4
ISBN-10: 1-59756-005-7
Library of Congress Control Number: 2005910834

CONTENTS

PREFACE

Since the mid-1970s, extraordinary advances in basic science, laryngology, and technology have resulted in dramatic improvements in our understanding of the human voice and in our ability to diagnose and treat voice disorders. Laryngeal electromyography (LEMG) is among the most important of these new developments.

Although laryngeal electromyography has been recognized since 1944 and important research regarding its application has been performed from the 1950s through the present day, its practical clinical importance has been appreciated only since the last decade of the twentieth century. Even now, many laryngologists do not have access to laryngeal electromyography, even though there are skilled electromyographers in their communities. Most electromyographers (neurologists, physiatrists, and others) have had no training in the study of laryngeal muscles and are reluctant initially to insert needles in laryngeal musculature. This book is written as an easy guide and quick reference for laryngologists, neurologists, physiatrists, and other potential electrophysiologists who are anxious to add laryngeal electromyography to their clinical armamentarium. Laryngeal electromyography can be performed by trained specialists in any of these fields, or collaboratively; but the availability of expert laryngeal electromyography is essential to accurate laryngologic diagnosis, and laryngeal electromyography should be available to any voice care team.

The first edition of this book covered most of the practical parts of laryngeal electromyography, as well as essential scientific information required to understand the procedure and its interpretation. The second edition has updated and expanded these topics and added new information on evidence-based research and on intraoperative monitoring. Every effort has been made to keep the book easily readable and useful for practicing clinicians in various specialties.

Robert T. Sataloff, M.D., D.M.A.

ABOUT THE AUTHORS

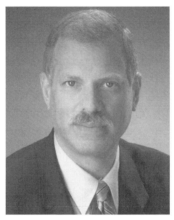

Robert Thayer Sataloff, M.D., D.M.A.

Dr. Sataloff is Professor of Otolaryngology-Head and Neck Surgery at Jefferson Medical College, Thomas Jefferson University in Philadelphia; Chairman of the Department of Otolaryngology–Head and Neck Surgery of Graduate Hospital; Adjunct Professor of Otorhinolaryngology–Head and Neck Surgery, University of Pennsylvania; on the faculty of the Academy of Vocal Arts; and Conductor of the Thomas Jefferson University Choir and Orchestra; and Director of the Voice Foundation's Annual Symposium on Care of the Professional Voice and the Chairman of the Board of Directors, American Institute for Voice and Ear Research. Dr. Sataloff is also a professional singer and singing teacher. He holds an undergraduate degree from Haverford College in Music Theory and Composition, graduated from Jefferson Medical College, Thomas Jefferson University, received a Doctor of Musical Arts in Voice Performance from Combs College of Music, and completed his residency in Oto-laryngology–Head and Neck Surgery and a Fellowship in Otology, Neurotology, and Skull Base Surgery at the University of Michigan. Dr. Sataloff is Chairman of the Board of Directors of the Voice Foundation and of the American Institute for Voice and Ear Research. He has also served as Chairman of the Board of Governors of Graduate Hospital, President of the International Association of Phono-surgery, President of the American Laryngological Association, and President of the Pennsylvania Academy of Otolaryngology–Head and Neck Surgery. He is Editor-in-Chief of the *Journal of Voice* and Editor-in-Chief of the *Ear, Nose and Throat Journal* and serves on the editorial review boards the *Journal of Singing, Medical Problems of Performing Artists,* and many major otolaryngology journals in the United States. Dr. Sataloff has written more than 600 publications, including 35 books. His medical practice is limited to care of the professional voice and to otology-neurotology-skull base surgery

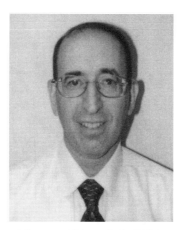

Steven Mandel, M.D.

Dr. Mandell is Clinical Professor of Neurology at Jefferson Medical College. He received his medical degree from Albert Einstein College of Medicine in Bronx, New York. He is president of Neurology and Neurophysiology Associates of Pennsylvania and New Jersey. His areas of interest include neuromuscular electrophysiology, minor head injury, peripheral nerve disorders, laryngeal electromyography, and disability medicine. He has co-edited three books, *Minor Head Injury*, *The Handbook of Neurology of the Lower Extremities*, and *Laryngeal Electromyography*, and has published more than 100 articles. Dr. Mandel is associate editor of the *Journal of Disability* and *Disability Medicine*. He is a frequent lecturer and has actively participated in community service organizations for adults and children with disabilities. Dr. Mandel is married to Heidi Mandel, doctor of podiatric medicine, and has three children, Jesse, Elisabeth, and David.

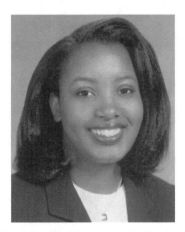

Yolanda D. Heman-Ackah, MD

Dr. Heman-Ackah is a laryngologist who specializes in professional voice care. She is board certified by the American Board of Oto-laryngology and is a fellow of the American Academy of Otolaryn-gology–Head and Neck Surgery. She received her Bachelor of Arts degree in Psychology and her Doctor of Medicine degree from Northwestern University as part of the Honors Program in Medical Education. Following her residency in otolaryngology–head and neck surgery at the University of Minnesota, she completed a fellowship in professional voice care and laryngology under the preceptorship of Robert T. Sataloff, MD, DMA in Philadelphia, PA. She then founded and was the director of the Voice Center at the University of Illinois at Chicago. Currently, she is in practice in association with Drs. Robert T. Sataloff, Karen M. Lyons, and John A. Tucker in Philadelphia, Pennsyvania. She is Assistant Professor in the Depart-ment of Otolaryngology–Head and Neck Surgery at Jefferson Med-ical College, Thomas Jefferson University in Philadelphia and is the National Medical Advisor for the Voice and Speech Trainer's Asso-ciation (VASTA). She has received awards and recognition for her research investigating the laryngeal chemoreflex, including an award from the American Academy of Otolaryngology–Head and Neck Surgery and research grants from the American Laryngological

Association and the American Larynoglogical Voice Research and Education Foundation. She has authored or co-authored numerous publications, including award-winning journal articles, book chapters, and this book. She is a member of the editorial board of the *Journal of Voice* and other medical journals, and she is actively involved in the Voice Foundation, the National Association of Teachers of Singing (NATS), the Voice and Speech Trainer's Association, the Latin Academy of Recording Arts and Sciences, and the National Academy of Recording Arts and Sciences.

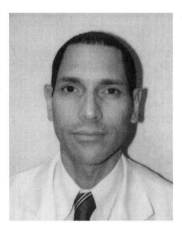

Ramon Mañon-Espaillat, MD, MA

Dr. Mañon-Espaillat is Clinical Professor of Neurology, Jefferson Medical College, Thomas Jefferson University. Dr. Mañon-Espaillat is also a Diplomate of the American Board of Psychiatry and Neurology, Diplomate of the American Board of Psychiatry and Neurology with added qualifications for Clinical Neurophysiology, Diplomate of the American Board of Clinical Neurophysiology, Diplomate of the American Association of Neuromuscular and Electrodiagnostic Medicine, and Diplomate of the American Board of Sleep Medicine. He has written numerous publications.

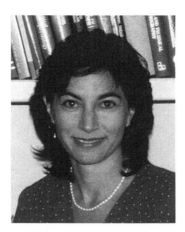

Mona Abaza, MD

Dr. Abaza received her undergraduate degree in biology from Pennsylvania State University and her medical degree from The Medical College of Pennsylvania in 1991. Her surgical training began at the University of Medicine and Dentistry of New Jersey in Newark, NJ followed by a two-year Intramural Research Training Award Fellowship at the National Institute on Deafness and Other Communication Disorders (National Institutes of Health in Bethesda, Md.). After leaving the NIH, she began her Otolaryngology–Head and Neck Surgery residency at the University of Texas Health Science Center in San Antonio. She then completed a fellowship in Laryngology/Professional Voice Care with Robert Sataloff, MD, DMA, at the American Institute for Ear and Voice Research in Philadelphia, Pennsylvania. Joining the University of Colorado Health Sciences Center, Department of Otolaryngology–Head and Neck Surgery as an Assistant Professor in 1999, she is currently Associate Residency Program Director. Dr. Abaza most recently opened the University of Colorado Hospital Voice Practice at the National Center for Voice and Speech at the Denver Center for Performing Arts, where she serves is medical director.

ACKNOWLEDGMENTS

The authors are indebted to Mary J. Hawkshaw for her editorial assistance and to Beth J. Luby and Helen M. Caputo for their invaluable help with preparation of the manuscript.

To Our Families

CHAPTER 1

Laryngeal Electromyography

Introduction and Overview

Laryngeal electromyography (LEMG) is a procedure that evaluates the integrity of the muscles and nerves of the larynx. The movements of the vocal folds are coordinated by the activities of the muscles of the larynx, the cartilages of the larynx, and the brain and nerves that supply the muscles of the larynx. Anatomy and physiology of the voice are discussed in Chapter 2. Details of the procedure and its clinical applications are introduced in this chapter and expanded upon in subsequent chapters; important points are summarized in Appendix I. Diagnostic LEMG is indicated in patients who have evidence of a movement disorder of the vocal folds. The purpose of diagnostic LEMG is to help elucidate the cause of these movement disorders and serve as a guide to diagnosis. Laryngeal motion abnormalities can be caused by joint dysfunction, muscular abnormalities, or central or peripheral neural disorders involving the larynx. Understanding the etiology of the motion abnormality is important in developing an effective treatment algorithm. LEMG has proven extremely helpful clinically, although evidence-based data confirming the usefulness of LEMG remain scarce (Appendix II). Movements of the vocal folds are coordinated by the activities of the muscles of the larynx, the cartilages of the larynx, and the brain and laryngeal nerves that supply the muscles of the larynx. Anatomy and physiology of the voice are discussed in Chapter 2.

PRINCIPLES OF AND INDICATIONS FOR DIAGNOSTIC LEMG

Diagnostic LEMG is performed to evaluate the integrity of the laryngeal neuromuscular system. LEMG takes advantage of the fact that nerves have an electrical signal that is transformed into a chemical signal at the neuromuscular junction. Electrodes are placed transcutaneously in the muscles of the larynx. The electrodes sense the electrical impulses within the muscle and convert them to visual and auditory signals that can be interpreted by the physician performing the procedure or an electrophysiologist.

LEMG PROCEDURE

LEMG is performed often as a diagnostic procedure, but it can also be used therapeutically to help guide the identification of the position of the laryngeal muscles for therapeutic injections and to monitor the activity of the laryngeal nerves during operative procedures. The procedure for LEMG for therapeutic and diagnostic indications involves the use of needle or hooked-wire electrodes via a percutaneous insertion technique. Intraoperative monitoring of the laryngeal nerves most commonly involves the use of surface electrodes, although needle and/or hooked-wire electrodes can also be used for this indication. Some otolaryngologists perform LEMG themselves. Neurologists physiatrists, or an electrophysiologist can also perform LEMG. The otolaryngologist's decision to perform LEMG with the help of other professionals depends on his or her level of comfort and expertise in interpreting electromyographic findings. Because neurologists, physiatrists, and electrophysiologists perform electromyography (EMG) on other neuromuscular systems on a daily basis, and because their professional training equips them with expertise in interpretation of complex neuromuscular electrical signals, many otolaryngologists prefer to have them assist in the interpretation of diagnostic LEMGs. Because the use of LEMG for botulinum toxin injections into laryngeal muscles requires a less sophisticated level of expertise in LEMG interpretation, often this procedure is performed solely by the otolaryngologist.

To perform LEMG, the patient is usually asked to lie down with the neck extended, a position that brings the larynx closer to the skin and aids the palpation of laryngeal landmarks for accurate insertion of the electrodes into the laryngeal muscles. As with all other sites of injections, the neck is cleansed first with alcohol. The insertion of the needles through the skin feels like a pinprick; the insertion into the muscles of the larynx may be almost free of sensation or may produce a mild stabbing sensation, similar to the sensation experienced when receiving an intramuscular injection. Local anesthetic can be given to prevent the pinprick sensation on the skin; however, injection of the anesthetic itself results in a pinprick sensation as well as a burning sensation and thus is not used routinely. Local anesthetic should not generally be given to reduce the sensations experienced during insertion of the electrodes into the muscles, as anesthesia may alter the electrical signals of the nerves and the muscles and confound the results; and it should not be given so a patient's ability to swallow and cough remains intact.

A surface or ground electrode is placed on the forehead, chest, or another part of the body away from the neck to help filter background electrical activity The electrode used in diagnostic LEMG is usually a needle electrode or a hooked-wire electrode that is inserted with the use of a needle. Because surface electrodes record electrical activity over a large surface area, they are not sensitive enough to provide accurate information about the small individual muscles in the larynx. Needle and hooked-wire electrodes sample electrical activity over a smaller surrounding area, and thus are better suited for recording the activity of the small intrinsic laryngeal muscles.

There are four pairs of muscle groups in the larynx: the thyroarytenoid (TA), the lateral cricoarytenoid (LCA), the posterior cricoarytenoid (PCA), and the cricothyroid (CT). There is also an unpaired interarytenoid muscle that is tested only rarely. The TA, PCA, and CT muscles are tested on each side routinely. Usually, testing of these three groups of muscles provides sufficient information about the integrity of the superior and recurrent laryngeal nerves and the muscles that they innervate for most clinical purposes. When equivocal results are obtained or when additional information is needed, the lateral cricoarytenoid and interarytenoid muscles may be tested as well. The needles are inserted through the skin and into the laryngeal muscles. The positions of the thyroid and cricoid cartilages are identified and the needle is passed through the cricothyroid membrane and in the direction of the muscle of interest. When the needle is positioned correctly, the patient is asked to perform laryngeal maneuvers (phonatory, respiratory, or swallowing) that require contraction of the muscle of interest and relative relaxation of the other muscles of the larynx. Testing of the cricothyroid muscle, for example, involves sliding from a low-pitched sound to a high-pitched sound. Testing the posterior cricoarytenoid muscle involves performing a forceful sniff. For the thyroarytenoid, lateral cricoarytenoid, and interarytenoid muscles, saying "/i/" produces the desired muscle activity. The anatomic distinction among these three muscles is that the thyroarytenoid muscle sits higher and more toward the middle of the larynx than does the lateral cricoarytenoid muscle; the lateral cricoarytenoid muscle sits laterally and posteriorly in the larynx; and, the interarytenoid muscle lies between the arytenoid cartilages and more posteriorly in the larynx than do the lateral cricoarytenoid and thyroarytenoid muscles. Differences of electrical activity in these muscles and in positioning of the needle for accurate insertion into each laryngeal muscle are discussed in Chapter 5. When the needle is in the correct position, the electrical signal seen on the oscilloscope and the auditory signal heard through the speakers will be increased with the appropriate phonatory, respiratory, or swallowing maneuver. If botulinum toxin is to be injected, it is injected through the EMG needle once the intended muscle is isolated. If LEMG is being performed for diagnostic purposes, the specific facets of the electrical signal are assessed as described briefly here and in detail in Chapters 4 and 5.

INTERPRETING LEMG RESULTS

Diagnostic LEMG involves the assessment of four main characteristics of the EMG signal: insertional activity, spontaneous activity, recruitment, and waveform morphology. The results of LEMG alone are not sufficient to establish a specific diagnosis. LEMG gives general information about the integrity of the motor units (the nerve fibers and their respective muscle fibers), the muscle, the nerve, and the neuromuscular junction and must be interpreted within the context of the clinical setting. A multitude of disease processes can produce damage to any of these structures. LEMG quantifies neuromuscular function and, sometimes, can give an indication of the chronicity of abnormal function. The etiology of the voice dysfunction is established on the basis of the history of the patient's voice dysfunction, the physical examination, imaging studies, laboratory studies, and results of LEMG and biopsies, as indicated by the suspected disease process.

Each of the factors investigated with LEMG provides an indication of the chronicity, the site of pathology, and the prognosis for recovery. Serial LEMGs can be performed to follow changes in nerve recovery or degeneration over time, allowing a better indication of the prognosis for recovery. In patients with paresis (weakness, hypomobility) or paralysis (complete nerve dysfunction, essentially immobility), the results of the LEMG may also help to guide subsequent voice therapy. If mild paresis is found, the patient should receive voice therapy aimed specifically at increasing the strength of the paretic muscle. In patients with moderate paresis and/or paralysis who may benefit from surgical procedures to enhance voice production, LEMG may aid in determining the nature and timing of the surgical procedure. If there is evidence of an ongoing neural degenerative process, surgery may be delayed until degeneration is complete or tailored to accommodate additional surgery as the disorder progresses. Similarly, if there is evidence of reinnervation, surgery may be delayed until maximal recovery has been achieved.

SUMMARY

LEMG is a procedure that evaluates the integrity of laryngeal nerves and muscles. It is particularly useful in differentiating disorders affecting the superior and recurrent laryngeal nerves from those affecting the laryngeal joints, neuromuscular junctions, or the muscles of the larynx. LEMG should be considered as an extension of the physical examination, not as an isolated laboratory procedure. LEMG abnormalities are interpreted within the broader clinical context and are used to assist in the diagnosis and treatment of vocal fold motion abnormalities.

CHAPTER 2

Anatomy and Physiology of the Voice

The anatomy of phonation is not limited to the larynx and neck. Virtually all body systems are involved, directly or indirectly, in voice production. This chapter provides a brief overview of the anatomy and physiology of the voice, with an emphasis on laryngeal anatomy relevant to electromyography. Readers interested in acquiring more than a clinically essential introduction are encouraged to consult other literature, including Sundberg's excellent text: *The Science of the Singing Voice*,[1] *Physiology of Phonation: A Review of Basic Mechanics*[2] by Scherer, and Sataloff's *Professional Voice: The Science and Art of Clinical Care,* Third Edition,[3] and the numerous references and suggested readings compiled in these sources.

ANATOMY

The *larynx* is essential to normal voice production. However, the vocal mechanism also includes the abdominal and back musculature, rib cage, lungs, pharynx, oral cavity, and nasal cavity. Each component performs an important function in voice production, although it is possible to produce voice without a larynx, for example, in patients who have undergone laryngectomy. Virtually all parts of the body play some role in voice production and may contribute to vocal dysfunction. Even something as remote as a sprained ankle may alter posture, thereby impairing abdominal, back, and thoracic muscle alignment and function and resulting in vocal inefficiency, weakness, voice fatigue, and hoarseness.[1-3]

The larynx is composed of four basic anatomic units: the skeleton, intrinsic muscles, extrinsic muscles, and mucosa. The most important parts of the laryngeal skeleton are the thyroid cartilage, the cricoid cartilage, and the paired arytenoid cartilages (Figure 2–1). These cartilages serve as the points of attachment for the intrinsic muscles of the larynx and rotate and/or tilt to move the vocal folds

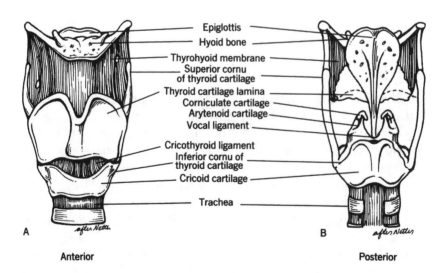

Epiglottis
Hyoid bone
Thyrohyoid membrane
Superior cornu of thyroid cartilage
Thyroid cartilage lamina
Corniculate cartilage
Arytenoid cartilage
Vocal ligament
Cricothyroid ligament
Inferior cornu of thyroid cartilage
Cricoid cartilage
Trachea

A   after Netter

B   after Netter

Anterior   Posterior

Fig 2-1. Cartilages of the larynx from anterior **(A)**, posterior **(B)**, superior *(continues)*

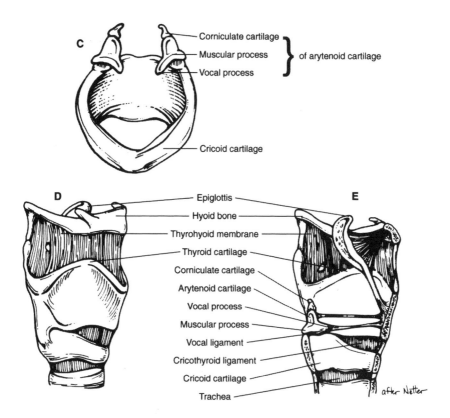

Fig 2-1. *(continued)* **(C)**, lateral **(D)**, and sagittal **(E)** perspectives show-ing the relationship of cricoid and arytenoid cartilages. (From Sataloff R, *Professional Voice: The Science and Art of Clinical Care.* 2nd ed. San Diego, Calif: Singular Publishing Group; 1997:112, with permission.)

as the intrinsic laryngeal muscles contract (Figure 2-2). The *thyro-arytenoid muscle* extends on each side from the vocal process of the arytenoid cartilage to the inside of the thyroid cartilage, just below and behind the thyroid notch, forming the body of the vocal folds (popularly called the "vocal cords"). The thyroarytenoid muscle has a medial and a lateral belly. The medial belly of the thyroary-tenoid muscle is also known as the vocalis muscle and is the deep-est layer of the vocal fold. The vocal folds act as the *oscillator* or *sound source* of the vocal tract. The space between the vocal folds is called the *glottis* and is used as an anatomic reference point.

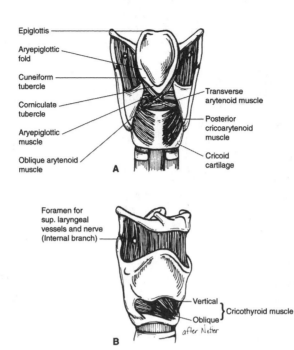

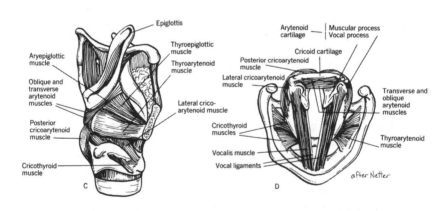

Fig 2-2. Intrinsic muscles of the larynx from posterior **(A)**, lateral **(B)**, internal **(C)**, and superior **(D)** perspectives. In the figures, the direction of the arrows suggests muscle actions, but may give a misleading impression of arytenoid motion. These drawings should not be misinterpreted as indicating that the arytenoid cartilage rotates around a vertical axis. The angle of the long axis of the cricoid facets does not permit some of the motion implied in this figure. However, the drawing still provides a useful conceptualization of the effect of individual intrinsic muscles, so long as the limitations are recognized. (From Sataloff R, *Professional Voice: The Science and Art of Clinical Care.* 2nd ed. San Diego. Calif: Singular Publishing Group; 1997:118, with permission.)

The "false vocal folds" are located above the true vocal folds and, unlike the true vocal folds, do not make contact or produce sound during normal speaking or singing.

The intrinsic muscles alter the position, shape, and tension of the vocal folds, through combinations of abduction, adduction, stretching, and condensing of the vocal folds (Figure 2-3). They are able to do so because the thyroid, cricoid, and arytenoid cartilages are connected by ligaments that allow changes in their relative angles and distances, thereby permitting alterations in the shape and tension of the vocal folds, which are suspended between them.

The arytenoid cartilages are thought of traditionally as being capable of rocking, rotating, and gliding, permitting complex vocal fold motion and alteration in the shape of the vocal fold edge (Figure 2-4). The thyroid cartilage tilts downward anteriorly along the axis of the cricothyroid joint to increase the tension in the vocal folds, and secondarily to slightly adduct them, when the cricothyroid muscle contracts. Because cricothyroid and cricoarytenoid joints are flexible, the positions of the cartilages with respect to each other change when the laryngeal skeleton is elevated or lowered. Such changes in vertical height of the laryngeal skeleton are controlled by the extrinsic laryngeal muscles, including the strap, the digastric stylohyoid, the mylohyoid, and geniohyoid muscles of the neck. When the angles and distances between the cartilages change, the resting lengths of the intrinsic muscles change. Gross changes in extrinsic muscle position interfere with fine control of the intrinsic muscles and, thus, affect the ability to maintain smooth vocal quality. Hence, classically trained singers are generally taught to use their extrinsic muscles to maintain the laryngeal skeleton at a relatively constant height, regardless of pitch. This control over the extrinsic laryngeal muscles allows one to overcome the natural tendency of the larynx to rise with ascending pitch and fall with descending pitch, thereby enhancing uniform quality throughout the vocal range.

All but one of the intrinsic muscles on each side of the larynx is innervated by the *recurrent laryngeal nerve*. Because each recurrent laryngeal nerve runs a long course from the neck into the chest (particularly on the left side) and then back up to the larynx (hence, the term "recurrent"), it is injured easily by trauma, neck surgery, and chest surgery. The cricothyroid muscle is innervated

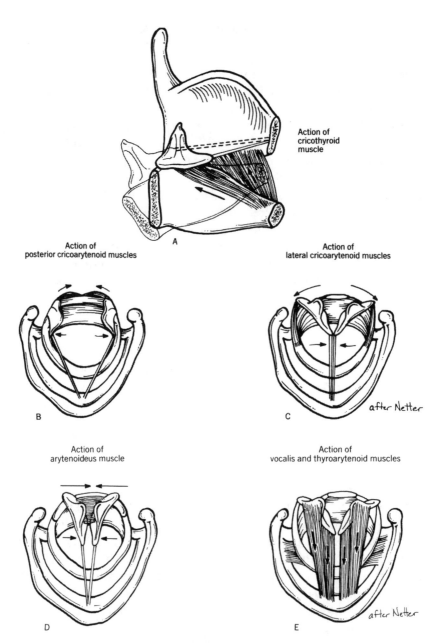

Action of
cricothyroid
muscle

Action of
posterior cricoarytenoid muscles

A

Action of
lateral cricoarytenoid muscles

after Netter

B

C

Action of
arytenoideus muscle

Action of
vocalis and thyroarytenoid muscles

after Netter

D

E

Fig 2-3. Action of the intrinsic muscles, including the cricothyroid **(A)**, posterior cricoarytenoid **(B)**, lateral cricoarytenoid **(C)**, interarytenoid **(D)**, and thyroarytenoid **(E)**. (From Sataloff R, *Professional Voice: The Science and Art of Clinical Care.* 2nd ed. San Diego: Singular Publishing Group; 1997:119, with permission.)

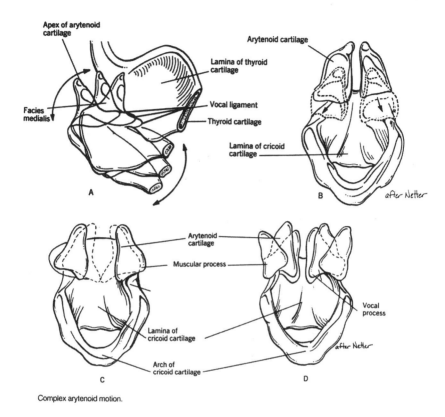

Complex arytenoid motion.

Fig 2–4. Complex arytenoid motion, showing response to cricothyroid contraction **(A)**, gliding **(B)**, rotating **(C)**, and rocking **(D)**. (From Gould WJ, Sataloff RT, Spiegel JR. *Voice Surgery.* St Louis, Mo: Mosby-Yearbook; 1993:164, with permission.)

by the ipsilateral *superior laryngeal nerve*, which is especially susceptible to viral and traumatic injury. The CT muscle controls increases in longitudinal tension that are important in projection and pitch control.

The neuroanatomy and neurophysiology of phonation are exceedingly complicated and are only partially understood. As the field of neurolaryngology continues to advance, a more thorough understanding of the subject will become increasingly important to clinicians.[4]

Mucosa

The soft tissues lining the larynx are much more complex than originally thought. The mucosa forms the thin, lubricated surface of the vocal folds that contact each other when the glottis is closed. Throughout most of the larynx, the mucosa consists of goblet cells, seromucinous glands, and pseudostratified-ciliated columnar epithelium designed for producing and handling mucous secretions, similar to the mucosa found throughout the respiratory tract. However, the mucosa overlying the superior and medial surfaces of the vocal folds is different. First, it is stratified squamous epithelium, better suited to withstand the repeated trauma of vocal fold contact. Second, there are no mucous glands or goblet cells within the vocal fold mucosa. However, the vocal folds are not simply muscle and ligament covered with mucosa. Rather, as described by Hirano,[5] they consist of five layers: epithelium; superficial, middle, and deep layers of lamina propria; and the vocalis muscle. Mechanically, the vocal fold's structure acts more like three layers, consisting of the *cover* (epithelium and superficial layer of the lamina propria), *transition* (intermediate and deep layers of the lamina propria, also commonly referred to as the vocal ligament), and *body* (the vocalis muscle) (Figure 2–5).

Innervation

The recurrent laryngeal nerve (RLN) and the superior laryngeal nerve (SLN) are branches of cranial nerve X, or the vagus nerve. The superior laryngeal nerve branches off the vagus high in the neck, just below the nodose ganglion. Each SLN divides into an internal branch and an external branch. The external branch supplies motor innervation to the cricothyroid muscle. An extension of this nerve may also supply motor and sensory innervation to the vocal folds. The internal branch is primarily responsible for sensory innervation of the mucosa at and above the level of the vocal folds in the glottic and supraglottic larynx, but it may also be responsible for some motor innervations of laryngeal muscles. The recurrent laryngeal nerves branch off the vagus in the upper chest or sometimes in the neck. On the left, the nerve usually loops

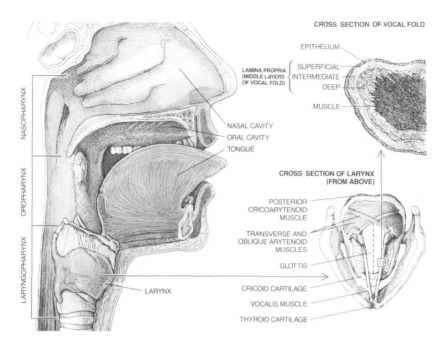

Fig 2–5. An overview of the larynx and vocal tract, showing the vocal folds and the region from which the vocal fold was sampled to obtain the cross-section showing the layered structure. (From Sataloff, RT. The human voice. *Scientific American.* 1992; 267:108–115, with permission.)

around the aortic arch at the level of the ligamentum arteriosum. On the right, it usually loops around the subclavian artery. This anatomic relationship is usually, but not always, present, and "nonrecurrent" recurrent nerves may be encountered. The RLN supplies motor innervation to all the intrinsic muscles of the larynx except the cricothyroid and sensation at and below the level of the vocal folds. There are interconnections between the superior and recurrent laryngeal nerves, particularly in the region of the interarytenoid muscle.

The motor fibers responsible for movement of the intrinsic laryngeal muscles originate in the nucleus ambiguus where they receive neural impulses from the motor cortex via the internal capsule. They travel laterally in the brainstem and exit the medulla in the groove between the olive and the pyramid. From there, the vagus exits the skull through the jugular foramen, with the superior laryngeal nerve branching off just below the nodose ganglion and the recurrent laryngeal nerve branching off in the chest.

The sensory fibers with the recurrent and superior laryngeal nerves synapse initially at the inferior vagal, or nodose ganglion. From there, sensory fibers ascend through the jugular foramen and enter the medulla. In the medulla, the fibers ascend to enter the nucleus of the tractus solitarius where synapses with the hypothalamus and the reticules formation occur to help mediate vagal reflexes.

Intrinsic Muscles

It is important to understand the function of individual laryngeal muscles for both laryngeal electromyography and voice care, in general. The muscles of primary functional importance are those innervated by the recurrent laryngeal nerves (thyroarytenoid, posterior cricoarytenoid, lateral cricoarytenoid, and interarytenoid or arytenoideus) and the superior laryngeal nerves (cricothyroid). These are the intrinsic laryngeal muscles. The thyroarytenoid muscle (TA) adducts, lowers, shortens, and thickens the vocal fold, rounding the vocal fold's edge (Figure 2-6). Thus, the cover and transition layers are effectively made more slack, while the body is stiffened. Adduction from vocalis contraction is active, particularly in the membranous segment of the vocal folds. Pitch is lowered from TA contraction as the vocal fold edge is shortened and thickened. The thyroarytenoid muscle originates anteriorly from the posterior surface of the thyroid cartilage and inserts into the lateral base of the arytenoid cartilages from the vocal process to the muscular process. More specifically, the superior bundles of the muscle insert into the lateral and inferior aspects of the vocal process and run primarily in a horizontal direction. The anteroinferior bundles insert into the anterolateral aspect of the arytenoid cartilage from its tip to an area lateral to the vocal process. The most medial fibers run parallel to the vocal ligament. There are also fibers that extend in a cephalad direction into the aryepiglottic fold. Anteriorly, the vertical organization of the muscle results in a twisted configuration of muscle fibers when the vocal folds are adducted.

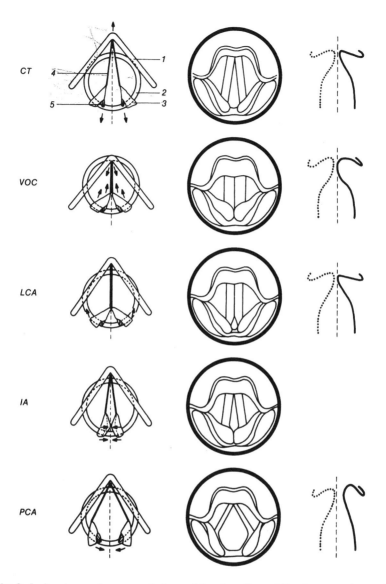

Fig 2-6. A schematic presentation of the function of the laryngeal muscles. The left column shows the location of the cartilages and the edge of the vocal folds when the laryngeal muscles are activated individually. The arrows indicate the direction of the force exerted. 1, thyroid cartilage; 2, cricoid cartilage; 3, arytenoid cartilage; 4, vocal ligament; 5, posterior cricoarytenoid ligament. The middle column shows the views from above. The right column illustrates contours of frontal sections at the middle of the membranous portion of the vocal fold. The dotted line illustrates the vocal fold position when no muscle is activated. CT, cricothyroid; VOC, vocalis; LCA, lateral cricoarytenoid; IA, interarytenoid; PCA, posterior cricoarytenoid. (From Hirano M. *Clinical Examination of Voice.* New York: Springer-Verlag; 1981:8, with permission.)

The thyroarytenoid is the third largest intrinsic muscle of the larynx and is divided into two compartments. The medial compartment, the vocalis muscle, contains a high percentage of slow-twitch muscle fibers. The lateral compartment has predominantly fast-twitch muscle fibers. One may infer that the medial compartment (vocalis) is specialized for prolonged phonation, while the lateral compartment (muscularis) is specialized for rapid vocal fold adduction, but these suppositions are unproven.

When the superior laryngeal nerves are activated, the cricothyroid muscles (CT) move the vocal folds into the paramedian position. The CT also lowers, stretches, elongates, and thins the vocal fold, stiffening all layers and sharpening the vocal fold's contour. It is the biggest intrinsic laryngeal muscle (although there are some anatomists who prefer to classify the CT as an extrinsic muscle). The cricothyroid muscle is largely responsible for increasing the longitudinal tension of the vocal fold edge, a very important factor in the control of pitch. This stretching of the vocal folds tends to increase vocal pitch. The cricothyroid muscle originates from the anterior and lateral portion of the arch of the cricoid cartilage and forms two bellies. The oblique belly inserts into the posterior half of the thyroid lamina and the anterior portion of the inferior cornu of the thyroid cartilage. The vertical (erect) belly inserts into the inferior border of the anterior lamina of the thyroid cartilage.

The lateral cricoarytenoid muscle (LCA) is a small muscle that adducts, lowers, elongates, and thins the vocal fold. All layers are stiffened, and the vocal fold's edge takes on a more angular or sharp contour. It originates on the upper lateral border of the cricoid cartilage and inserts into the anterior lateral surface of the muscular process of the arytenoid.

The interarytenoid muscle (IA), also called the arytenoideus, is a medium-size intrinsic muscle that primarily adducts the vocal process of the vocal fold. It is particularly important in providing medial compression to close the posterior glottis. It has relatively little effect on the stiffness of the membranous portion of the vocal fold. The interarytenoid muscle consists of transverse and oblique fibers. The transverse fibers originate from the lateral margin of one arytenoid and insert into the lateral margin of the contralateral arytenoid. The oblique also originate from the base of one arytenoid and insert into the apex of the contralateral arytenoid cartilage.

The posterior cricoarytenoid (PCA) muscle abducts, elevates, elongates, and thins the vocal fold by rocking the arytenoid cartilages posterolaterally. All layers are stiffened, and the edge of the vocal fold is rounded. It is the second largest intrinsic muscle. It originates over a broad area of the posterolateral portion of the cricoid lamina and inserts onto the posterior surface of the muscular process of the arytenoid cartilage, forming a short tendon that covers the cranial aspect of the muscular process.

The intrinsic laryngeal muscles are skeletal muscles. All skeletal muscles are composed primarily of three types of fibers. Type I fibers are highly resistant to fatigue, contract slowly, and utilize aerobic (oxidative) metabolism. They have low glycogen levels, high levels of oxidative enzymes, and are relatively small in diameter. Type IIA fibers use oxidative metabolism primarily but contain high levels of both oxidative enzymes and glycogen. They contract rapidly but are also fatigue-resistant. Type IIB fibers are the largest in diameter. They utilize anaerobic glycolysis primarily, and contain a high percentage of glycogen and relatively few oxidative enzymes. They contract very quickly, but fatigue easily.

The fiber distribution of laryngeal muscles differs from that of most larger skeletal muscles. Elsewhere, muscle fiber diameters are fairly constant, ranging between 60 and 80 microns. In laryngeal muscles, there is considerably more variability,[6,7] and fiber diameters vary between 10 and 100 microns, with an average diameter of 40 to 50 microns. Laryngeal muscles have a higher proportion of Type IIA fibers than most other muscles. The thyroarytenoid and lateral cricothyroid muscles are particularly specialized for rapid contraction. The other laryngeal muscles, in general, appear to have fiber distributions and variations that make them particularly well-suited to rapid contraction with fatigue resistance.[8] In addition, many laryngeal motor units have multiple innervations. There appear to be approximately 20 to 30 muscle fibers per motor unit in a human cricothyroid muscle,[9] suggesting that the motor unit size of this laryngeal muscle is similar to that of extraocular and facial muscles.[10] In the human thyroarytenoid muscle, 70% to 80% of muscle fibers have two or more motor endplates.[11]

Some fibers have as many as 5 motor endplates. Only 50% of cricothyroid and lateral cricoarytenoid fibers have multiple endplates, and multiple innervation is even less common in the posterior cricoarytenoid (5%). It is still not known whether some muscle fibers can be part of more than one motor unit (ie, receive motor end plates from more than one motor neuron).[8]

Extrinsic Muscles

The extrinsic laryngeal musculature maintains the position of the larynx in the neck. This group of muscles includes primarily the strap muscles, but also the digastric, mylohyoid, stylohyoid, and geniohyoid muscles. As raising or lowering the larynx may alter the tension or angle between laryngeal cartilages, thereby changing the resting lengths of the intrinsic muscles, the extrinsic muscles are critical in maintaining a stable laryngeal skeleton. In the Western classically trained singer, the extrinsic muscles maintain the larynx in a relatively constant vertical position throughout the pitch range. Training of the extrinsic musculature results in vibratory symmetry of the vocal folds, producing regular periodicity. This contributes to what the listener perceives as a "trained" sound.

The extrinsic muscles may be divided into those below the hyoid bone (infrahyoid muscles) and those above the hyoid bone (suprahyoid muscles). The *infrahyoid muscles* include the thyrohyoid, sternothyroid, sternohyoid, and omohyoid. The *thyrohyoid muscle* originates obliquely on the thyroid lamina and inserts into the lower border of the greater cornu of the hyoid bone. Contraction brings the thyroid cartilage closer to the hyoid bone, especially anteriorly, thereby, raising the position of the larynx in the neck. The *sternothyroid muscle* originates from the first costal cartilage and posterior aspect of the manubrium of the sternum. It inserts obliquely on the thyroid cartilage. Contraction lowers the thyroid cartilage. The *sternohyoid muscle* originates from the clavicle and posterior surface of the manubrium of the sternum, inserting into the lower edge of the body of the hyoid bone. Contraction lowers the hyoid bone. The inferior belly of the omohyoid originates from the upper surface of the scapula and inserts into the intermediate tendon of the *omohyoid muscle*. The superior belly extends from the intermediate tendon to the greater cornu of the hyoid bone.

The omohyoid muscle pulls down the hyoid bone, thus tending to lower it.

The *suprahyoid muscles* include the digastric, mylohyoid, geniohyoid, and stylohyoid. The posterior belly of the *digastric muscle* originates from the mastoid process and inserts into the intermediate tendon, which connects to the hyoid bone. The anterior belly originates from the inferior aspect of the mandible near the symphysis and inserts into the intermediate tendon. The anterior belly pulls the hyoid bone anteriorly and also raises it, and the posterior belly pulls the hyoid bone posteriorly while raising it. The *mylohyoid muscle* originates from the inner aspect of the mandible (mylohyoid line) and inserts into a midline raphe with fibers from the opposite side. It raises the hyoid bone and pulls it anteriorly. The *geniohyoid muscle* originates from the mental spine at the mental symphysis of the mandible and inserts on the anterior surface of the body of the hyoid bone. It raises the hyoid bone and pulls it anteriorly. The *stylohyoid muscle* originates from the styloid process and inserts into the body of the hyoid bone. It raises the hyoid bone and pulls it posteriorly. Coordinated interaction among the extrinsic laryngeal muscles is needed to control the vertical position of the larynx, as well as other conditions, such as laryngeal tilt.

The Supraglottic Vocal Tract

The supraglottic vocal tract includes the oral cavity, pharynx, nasal cavity, and possibly the sinuses which together, function as resonators and shape the sound quality produced by the vocal folds. Minor alterations in the configuration of these structures may produce substantial changes in voice quality. The hypernasal speech typically associated with a cleft palate and/or the hyponasal speech characteristic of severe adenoid hypertrophy are obvious. However, mild edema from an upper respiratory tract infection, mild pharyngeal scarring from tonsillectomy, or muscle tension changes produce less obvious sound alterations. These are immediately recognizable to a trained vocalist or to the astute critic, but they may elude the unsuspecting physician.

Abdomen and Thorax

In singing and speaking, the lungs supply a constant stream of air that passes between the vocal folds and provides power for voice production. Singers often are thought of as having "big chests." Actually, the primary respiratory difference between trained and untrained singers is not increased total lung capacity, as popularly assumed. Rather, the trained singer learns to use a higher proportion of the air in his or her lungs, thereby decreasing residual volume and increasing respiratory efficiency.[12]

The abdominal musculature is the so-called "support" of the speaking and singing voice, although singers commonly refer to this support mechanism as the "diaphragm." The function of the diaphragm muscle in singing and speaking is complex and somewhat variable from singer to singer (or from actor to actor). The diaphragm generates primarily inspiratory force. Although the abdomen can also perform this function in some situations,[13] it is primarily an expiratory force generator. Interestingly, the diaphragm is coactivated by some performers during singing and appears to play an important role in fine regulation of singing.[14]

Both the lungs and rib cage generate passive expiratory forces under many common circumstances. Passive inspiratory forces also occur. Active respiratory muscles working in concert with passive forces include the intercostal, abdominal wall, back muscles, and the diaphragm. The principal muscles of inspiration are the diaphragm and external intercostal muscles. Accessory muscles of inspiration include the pectoralis major; pectoralis minor; serratus anterior; subclavius; sternocleidomastoid; anterior, medial, and posterior scalenus; serratus posterior and superior; latissimus dorsi; and levatores costarum. During quiet respiration, expiration is largely passive. Many of the muscles used for active expiration are also employed in "support" for singing and acting. Muscles of active expiration either raise the intra-abdominal pressure, forcing the diaphragm upward; or lower the ribs or sternum to decrease the dimension of the thorax; or both. They include the internal intercostals, which stiffen the intercostal spaces and pull the ribs down; the transversus thoracis, subcostal muscles, and serratus posterior inferior, all of which pull the ribs down; and the quadratus lumborum, which depresses the lowest rib. In addition, the latissimus dorsi is capable of compressing the lower portion of the rib cage and can act as a muscle of expiration as well as a muscle of inspiration.

The above muscles all participate in active expiration (and support). However, the *primary* muscles of active expiration are the abdominal muscles. They include the external oblique, internal oblique, rectus abdominus, and transversus abdominus. The external oblique is a flat, broad muscle located on the side and front of the lower chest and abdomen. Upon contraction, it pulls the lower ribs down and raises the abdominal pressure by displacing abdominal contents inward. It is one of the most important muscles for support for both speaking and singing. It should be noted that this muscle is strengthened by a combination of trunk flexion and twisting and similar exercises, but is not developed effectively by traditional or curl sit-ups. Appropriate strengthening exercises of the external oblique muscles are often inappropriately neglected in voice training. The internal oblique is a flat muscle located on the side and front wall of the abdomen. It lies deep to the external oblique. When contracted, the internal oblique drives the abdominal wall inward and lowers the lower ribs. The rectus abdominus runs parallel to the midline of the abdomen, originating from the xiphoid process of the sternum and the fifth, sixth, and seventh costal cartilages. It inserts into the pubis. It is encased in the fibrous abdominal aponeurosis. Contraction of the rectus abdominus also forces the abdominal contents inward and lowers the sternum and ribs. The transversus abdominus is a broad muscle located under the internal oblique on the side and front walls of the abdomen. Contraction of the transverse abdominus compresses the abdominal contents, thus increasing intra-abdominal pressure.

PHYSIOLOGY OF THE VOICE

The physiology of voice production is complex. Volitional production of voice begins in the cerebral cortex (Figure 2–7). The command for vocalization involves interaction among the centers for speech and other areas of the brain. For singing and speech emotion, directives must be integrated with information from the brain centers for musical and artistic expression. The "idea" of the planned vocalization is conveyed to the precentral gyrus in the

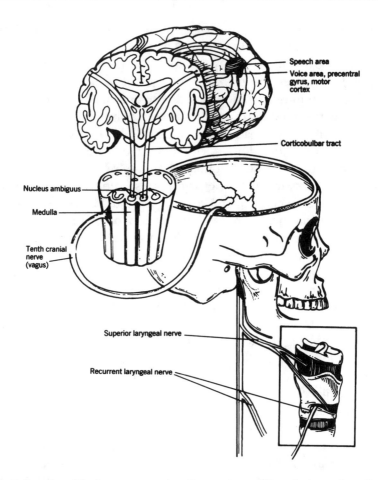

Fig 2–7. Simplified summary of pathway for volitional phonation.(From Gould WJ, Sataloff RT, Spiegel JR. *Voice Surgery.* St. Louis, Mo: Mosby-Yearbook; 1993:166, with permission.)

motor cortex, which transmits another set of instructions to the motor nuclei in the brainstem and spinal cord. These areas send out the complicated messages necessary for coordinated activity of the larynx, thoracic and abdominal musculature, and vocal tract articulators via the peripheral nervous system. Additional refinement of motor activity is provided by the extrapyramidal and autonomic nervous systems. These impulses combine to produce a sound that is transmitted not only to the ears of the listener, but also to those of the speaker or singer. Auditory feedback is transmitted from the ear to the brainstem to the cerebral cortex, and adjustments are made to permit the vocalist to match the sound produced with the sound intended, taking into account the acoustic properties of the environment. There is also tactile feedback from the throat and muscles involved in phonation that is believed to help in the fine-tuning of vocal output, although the mechanism and role of tactile feedback are not fully understood. In many trained singers and speakers, the ability to use tactile feedback effectively is cultivated as a result of expected interference with auditory feedback by ancillary noise such as an orchestra or band.

The *supraglottic vocal tract* includes the pharynx, tongue, palate, oral cavity, nose, and other structures. Together, they act as a *resonator* and are largely responsible for vocal quality or timbre and the perceived character of all speech sounds. The vocal folds themselves produce only a buzzing sound. During the course of vocal training for singing, acting, or healthy speaking, changes occur not only in the larynx, but also in the motion, control, and shape of the supraglottic vocal tract.

The *infraglottic vocal tract* serves as the *power source* for the voice. This includes the lungs, chest, abdomen, and back. Singers and actors refer to the entire power source complex as their "support" or "diaphragm." Actually, the anatomy of support for phonation is especially complicated and not completely understood. Yet, it is quite important because deficiencies in support are frequently responsible for voice dysfunction.

Phonation requires interaction of the power source, oscillator, and resonator. The voice may be likened to a brass instrument such as a trumpet. Power is generated by the chest, abdomen, and back musculature, producing a high-pressure airstream. The trumpeter's lips open and close against the mouthpiece producing a buzz similar to the sound produced by the vocal folds. This sound then passes through the trumpet, which has resonance characteristics that shape the sound we associate with trumpet music. The non-mouthpiece portion of a brass instrument is analogous to the supraglottic vocal tract.

During phonation, rapid, complex adjustments of the infraglottic musculature are necessary because the resistance changes almost continuously as the glottis closes, opens, and changes shape

(Figure a–j). At the beginning of each phonatory cycle, the vocal folds are approximated—that is, the glottis is obliterated. This permits infraglottic pressure to build up, typically to a level of about 7 cm of water for conversational speech. At this point, the vocal folds are convergent and there is no airflow. The subglottic pressure pushes the vocal folds progressively farther apart from the bottom up (Figures 2–8a and 2–8b) until a space develops (Figure 2–8c) and air begins to flow. A Bernoulli force is created by the air as it passes between the vocal folds, and the elasticity of the vocal folds results in closure of the lower portion of the glottis almost immediately (Figures 2–8d–g), even while the upper edges are still separating. The upper portion of the vocal folds has strong elastic properties, which tend to make the vocal folds snap back to the midline. This force becomes more dominant as the upper edges are stretched farther apart and as the force of the airstream diminishes because of approximation of the lower edges of the vocal folds. Therefore, the upper portion of the vocal folds return to the midline (Figures 2–8h and 2–8i), completing the glottic cycle. Subglottal pressure then increases again (Figure 2–8j), and the events are repeated. The frequency of vibration (number of cycles of openings and closings per second, measured in hertz [Hz]) is dependent on the air pressure and on mechanical properties of the vocal folds, which are regulated by the laryngeal muscles.

Frequency of phonation corresponds closely with perception of pitch. Under most circumstances, as the vocal folds are thinned and stretched, and air pressure is increased, the frequency of air pulse emission increases and pitch goes up. In understanding this myoelastic-aerodynamic mechanism of phonation, it is important to note that the vocal folds not only emit pulses of air (rather than vibrating like strings), but that there also is a vertical phase difference. That is, the lower portion of the vocal folds begins to open and close before the upper portion. The rippling displacement of the vocal fold's cover produces a mucosal wave that can be examined clinically under stroboscopic light. If this complex motion is impaired, hoarseness or other changes in voice quality may result. The sound produced by the vibrating vocal folds and modified by the vocal tract is a complex tone containing a fundamental frequency and many overtones, or higher harmonic partials. The amplitude of the partials decreases uniformly at approximately

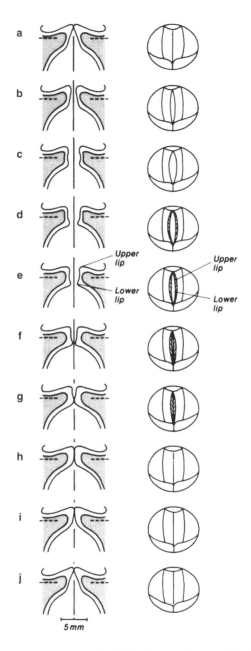

a

b

c

d

e — Upper lip / Lower lip (left); Upper lip / Lower lip (right)

f

g

h

i

j

5 mm

Fig 2-8. Vibration of the vocal folds is shown, in a vertical cross-section through the middle part of the vocal fold, during the production of a single sound. The perspective is from the front of the larynx. Before the process starts **(a)**, the folds are together. They separate as air is forced upward through the trachea **(b–g)** and then come together again as the sound ceases **(h)**.

12 dB per octave. Interestingly, the spectrum of the voice source is about the same in both untrained singers and speakers and trained singers and speakers. However, voice quality differences occur as the voice source signal passes through the supraglottic vocal tract (Figure 2–9).

The pharynx, oral cavity, and nasal cavity act as a series of interconnected resonators, more complex than, but analogous to, a trumpet or other single resonator. As with other resonators, some frequencies are attenuated, while others are enhanced. Enhanced or resonance frequencies are equated with higher relative amplitudes. Sundberg has shown that the vocal tract has four or five important resonance frequencies, called formants.[1] The presence of formants alters the uniformly sloping voice source spectrum, creating peaks at formant frequencies. These alterations of the voice source spectral envelope are responsible for distinguishable sounds of speech and song. Formant frequencies are established by vocal tract shape, which can be altered by laryngeal, pharyngeal, and oral cavity musculature.

While overall vocal tract length and shape are fixed individually and determined by age and sex (females and children have shorter vocal tracts and higher formant frequencies than those of males), mastering adjustment of vocal tract shape is fundamental to voice training. Although the formants differ for different vowels, one resonance frequency, known as the singer's formant, has received particular attention.[1] The singer's formant occurs in the vicinity of 2300 to 3200 Hz for all vowel spectra and appears to be responsible for the "ring" in a trained singer's or speaker's voice. The ability to hear a trained voice clearly even over a loud choir or orchestra is dependent primarily on the presence of the singer's formant.[1] Interestingly, there is little or no significant difference in maximum vocal intensity between a trained singer and an untrained singer. The singer's formant also contributes significantly to the difference in timbre among voice categories, occurring in basses at about 2400 Hz, baritones at 2600 Hz, tenors at 2800 Hz, mezzo-sopranos at 2900 Hz, and sopranos at 3200 Hz. It is much less prominent in high soprano singing.

Control mechanisms for two vocal characteristics, fundamental frequency and intensity, are particularly important. Fundamental frequency, which corresponds to pitch, can be altered by changing

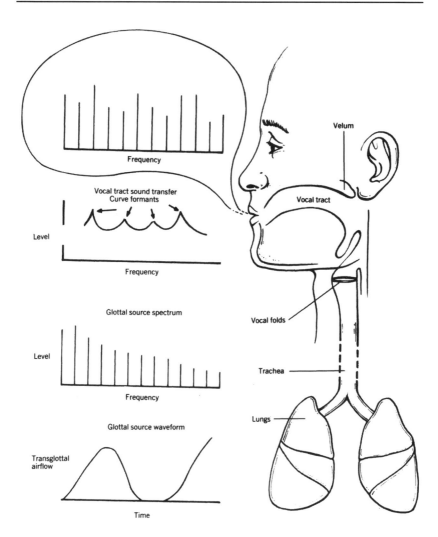

Fig 2-9. Determinants of the spectrum of a vowel (oral-output signal). (From Sataloff R, *Professional Voice: The Science and Art of Clinical Care.* 2nd ed. San Diego, Calif: Singular Publishing Group; 1997:168, with permission.)

either the air pressure or the mechanical properties of the vocal folds, although the latter is more efficient under most conditions. Contracting the cricothyroid muscle makes the thyroid cartilage pivot, increasing the distance between the thyroid and arytenoid cartilages and consequently stretching the vocal folds. This increases the surface area exposed to subglottal pressure and makes the air pressure more effective in opening the vocal folds. In addition, the elastic fibers of the vocal folds are stretched, making them more efficient at snapping back together. Hence, the cycles shorten and repeat more frequently, and the fundamental frequency (and pitch) rises. Other muscles, including the thyroarytenoid, also contribute. Raising the pressure of the airstream also tends to increase fundamental frequency, a phenomenon for which singers must compensate. Otherwise, pitch would increase with volume.

Vocal intensity, which corresponds to loudness, depends on the degree to which the glottal wave excites the air in the vocal tract. Raising the air pressure creates greater amplitude of vocal fold vibration and, consequently, increased vocal intensity. However, it is not vibration of the vocal folds but rather the sudden cessation of airflow that is responsible for establishing acoustic vibration in the vocal tract and controlling intensity. This is similar to the acoustic vibration created by clapping hands or, more accurately, buzzing lips. In the larynx, the sharper the flow cutoff, the more intense the sound. In fact, great vocal intensity is marked primarily by a steeper closing phase of the glottal wave, achieved by both higher air pressure and biomechanical vocal fold changes that increase glottal resistance to airflow.

Assessing an individual's ability to optimize adjustments of air pressure and glottal resistance may be helpful in identifying and correcting voice dysfunction. If high subglottic pressure is combined with high adductory vocal fold force, glottal airflow and the amplitude of the voice source fundamental frequency are low. This is called *pressed phonation* and can be measured clinically through flow glottography. If adductory forces are so weak that the vocal folds do not make contact, the glottis becomes inefficient and the voice source fundamental frequency is low. This is known as *breathy phonation. Flow phonation* is characterized by relatively low subglottic pressure and low adductory force. These conditions increase the dominance of the fundamental frequency of the voice source. Sundberg has shown that the amplitude of the fundamental frequency can be increased by 15 dB or more when changing from pressed phonation to flow phonation.[1] If a patient habitually uses pressed phonation, considerable effort will be required to achieve loud voicing. The muscle patterns and force often used to compensate for this laryngeal inefficiency may cause vocal damage. Such muscle hyperfunction shows distinctive patterns on LEMG that are distinguished easily from neuromuscular pathology.

SUMMARY

Anatomy and physiology of phonation are complex, fascinating topics. This chapter has emphasized facts of particular clinical importance as they relate to neurolaryngeal function. Assessment of laryngeal function is only one aspect in the evaluation of voice dysfunction. The entire vocal mechanism should be evaluated in all patients with dysphonia.

REFERENCES

1. Sundberg J. *The Science of the Singing Voice.* DeKalb: Northern Illinois University Press; 1987:1-216.
2. Scherer RS. Physiology of phonation: a review of basic mechanics. In: Ford CN, Bless DM, eds. *Phonosurgery.* New York, NY: Raven Press; 1991:77-93.
3. Sataloff RT. Clinical anatomy and physiology of the voice. In: Sataloff RT, *Professional Voice: The Science and Art of Clinical Care.* 3rd ed. San Diego, Calif, Plural Publishing; 2005.
4. Garrett JD, Larson CR. Neurology of the laryngeal system. In: Ford CN, Bless DM, eds. *Phonosurgery.* New York, NY: Raven Press; 1991: 43-76.
5. Hirano M. Phonosurgery: basic and clinical investigations. *Otologia (Fukuoka).* 1975;21:239-442.
6. Brooke MH, Engle WK. The histographic analysis of human muscle biopsies with regard to fibre types. Part 1. Adult male and female. *Neurology.* 1969;19:221-233.
7. Sadeh M, Kronenberg J., Gaton E. Histochemistry of human laryngeal muscles. *Cell Molec Biol.* 1981;27:643-648.
8. Lindestad P. *Electromyographic and Laryngoscopic Studies of Normal and Disturbed Vocal Function.* Stockholm, Sweden: Huddinge University;1994:1-12.
9. English ET, Blevins CE. Motor units of laryngeal muscles. *Arch Otolaryngol.* 1969;89:778-784.

10. Faaborg-Andersen K. Electromyographic investigation of intrinsic laryngeal muscles in humans. *Acta Physiol Scand.* 1957; 41(suppl 140); 1–149.

11. Rossi G, Cortesina G. Morphological study of the laryngeal muscles in man: insertions and courses of the muscle fibers, motor end-plates and proprioceptors. *Acta Otolaryngol* (Stockh). 1965;59:575–592.

12. Gould WJ, Kamura H. Static lung volumes in singers. *Ann Otol Rhinol Laryngol.* 1973;82:89–95.

13. Hixon TJ, Hoffman C. Chest wall shape during singing. In: Lawrence V, ed. *Transcripts of the Seventh Annual Symposium, Care of the Professional Voice.* New York, NY: The Voice Foundation; 1978;1: 9–10.

14. Sundberg J, Leanderson R, von Euler C. Activity relationship between diaphragm and cricothyroid muscles. *J Voice.* 1989;3(3):225–232.

CHAPTER 3

Vocal Fold Hypomobility

Normally, the vocal folds move to open the glottis for respiration, and to close the glottis for airway protection and phonation. Movement may be impaired by neurologic or mechanical conditions. Because symptoms and signs of hypomobility may be similar regardless of the etiology of the movement disorder, it is essential to diagnose causal conditions accurately in order to optimize treatment.

SYMPTOMS OF VOCAL FOLD HYPOMOBILITY

Patients with movement disorders of the larynx typically have complaints of hoarseness, breathiness, vocal fatigue, decreased range, vocal instability, decreased projection, and occasionally problems with shortness of breath, swallowing, or choking while eating or drinking. A patient who has decreased vocal fold mobility usually will experience hoarseness, breathiness, and/or vocal fatigue. Hoarseness is sometimes perceived because of abnormal strain in the supraglottic pharyngeal, and/or extrinsic laryngeal muscles as the patient tries to adduct the vocal folds. This excess muscle tension may sometimes result in false vocal fold phonation (dysphonia plica ventricularis), which has a more raspy or hoarse quality than phonation produced by the true vocal folds. Usually, a breathy voice quality is the result of air escaping through incompletely closed vocal folds. In most cases of paresis and paralysis, the opposite (normal) vocal fold attempts to compensate for the incomplete mobility of the affected vocal fold by closing not only to the midline, but past the midline to meet the weakened vocal fold. If the normal vocal fold is unable to compensate completely, a glottic gap will occur with vocalization. Subglottic air pressure decreases as air leaks past the incompetent glottis, resulting in a lower glottal flow rate and turbulent airflow at and above the level of the vocal folds. The turbulent airflow through the glottic gap results in decreased periodicity of the glottic cycle that is perceived as hoarseness and/or breathiness. To maintain a normal volume, the patient must increase the subglottic pressure and pulmonary effort to compensate for the inefficiency at the level of the glottis. As a result, prolonged phonation becomes more effortful, especially as the patient strains to compensate. Many patients describe this sensation as vocal fatigue.

The primary function of the vocal folds is to protect the lungs and the trachea from aspiration of food and liquids during swallowing. If vocal fold hypomobility limits the ability of the vocal folds to close completely during swallowing, aspiration may occur. If the sensation in the larynx and trachea is normal, then the patient experiences choking or coughing each time food or liquid is aspirated. If the sensory nerves are also damaged, then aspiration may occur without signs of choking or coughing, a phenomenon sometimes referred to as "silent aspiration." If impaired vocal fold mobility is secondary to nerve dysfunction and the sensory portions of the nerve are affected by the same problem that is limiting the motor function of the nerve, then hypesthesia or anesthesia may be present. It is also possible for decreased sensation (hypesthesia or anesthesia) to be present from independent, unrelated nerve abnormalities such as postherpetic neuropathy, diabetic neuropathy, or other causes.

DIAGNOSIS OF VOCAL FOLD
HYPOMOBILITY OR IMMOBILITY

A patient who has voice complaints generally is evaluated by an otolaryngologist or laryngologist. A complete history of the voice disorder is obtained. The physical examination will include a complete evaluation of all structures of the head and neck, including the ears, nose, oral cavity, face, pharynx, larynx, and neck to evaluate for multiple cranial nerves neuropathies and other abnormalities that can affect more than one organ system in the head and neck.

Examination of the larynx and the hypopharynx is performed initially with a light and mirror. On examination with the mirror, the physician may observe gross movement disorders of the larynx. Because subtleties in movement disorders are difficult to assess with mirror examination alone, flexible and/or rigid laryngoscopy should be performed to allow better examination of the mobility and structure of the vocal folds.

The flexible laryngoscope allows for evaluation of the larynx in its natural position, without the distortion that sometimes occurs with pulling the tongue forward for mirror and rigid telescopic examinations. By viewing the larynx in its natural posture, changes in laryngeal muscle tension while the patient is talking or singing can be assessed. During the flexible laryngoscopic examination, the patient is asked to perform several phonatory and swallowing maneuvers to assess fully the laryngeal biomechanics. These include various tasks of talking, singing, whistling, and swallowing. While the patient is performing these maneuvers, the otolaryngologist/laryngologist is evaluating the mobility of the vocal folds. The patient is asked also to perform several phonatory tasks that require stretching and lengthening of the vocal folds. These tasks may include counting at several different pitches and/or sliding from a low pitch to a high pitch while saying the sound /i/. If there is a primary problem in the superior laryngeal nerve, it may be shown as an inability to stretch and lengthen the vocal fold fully with high-pitched phonation. If only one of the cricothyroid muscles is paretic, this may be evident on examination as a decreased ability to lengthen the vocal fold on the side of the weakness; if the weakness is severe, there can be a tilt of the larynx toward the side of the weakened superior laryngeal nerve.

If there are problems with both superior laryngeal nerves, there will be limitations in the ability to produce a high pitch and in the ability to stretch the vocal folds on both sides. This diagnosis may be somewhat difficult to make, especially if both nerves are injured to the same degree. If there is some function in the nerves, then both vocal folds will stretch to the same limited degree, making the ability to discern subtle abnormalities difficult for the examiner. The finding of bilaterally decreased recruitment on LEMG is particularly helpful in confirming this diagnosis when it is suspected.

Often with superior laryngeal nerve paresis, there is also an abnormality in the ability of the vocal fold on the affected side to adduct. This results in sluggish movement of the vocal fold on the side of the larynx with the superior laryngeal nerve paresis and is seen best when the patient engages in vocal maneuvers that involve rapid movement of the vocal folds. These vocal fold maneuvers involve performing such repetitive tasks as saying /i/-/hi/, alternating a quick sniff with saying /i/, and/or saying /pa/-/ta/-/ka/, repeatedly until the patient begins to fatigue. Because these vocal maneuvers involve rapid movement of the vocal folds, they easily elicit subtle differences in vocal fold motion.

If the recurrent laryngeal nerve is injured, there may be abnormalities in adduction (bringing the vocal folds toward the midline) or abduction (opening the vocal folds). The recurrent laryngeal nerve supplies both the posterior cricoarytenoid muscle, the primary vocal fold abductor, and the thyroarytenoid, interarytenoid, and lateral cricoarytenoid muscles, the primary vocal fold adductors. Abnormalities in adduction are evaluated by the same maneuvers described above. Differentiating dysfunction involving the superior laryngeal nerve versus the recurrent laryngeal nerve when sluggish adduction is seen can be difficult. In general, if the problem is with the superior laryngeal nerve alone, one should also see problems with stretching the vocal folds. If the problem involves the recurrent laryngeal nerve, abnormalities should be seen with adduction and usually with abduction, but not with stretching the vocal folds.

Abnormalities in abduction frequently are evaluated by having the patient sniff and whistle. Both of these maneuvers require that the vocal folds open briskly. If the recurrent laryngeal nerve is injured at its insertion into the posterior cricoarytenoid muscle, the vocal fold will have isolated problems with abduction. If the injury to the nerve occurs at the level of the thyroarytenoid or lateral cricoarytenoid muscles, there will be isolated abnormalities in vocal fold adduction. If there is a problem with the nerve at any point before it enters the larynx, there may be abnormalities in both abduction and adduction. It has been observed, however, that in cases of paresis, "normal" laryngeal muscles can fatigue, resulting in an apparent weakness on physical examination. Thus, these are merely guidelines to identifying the paretic laryngeal nerve on physical examination. When asymmetries are found on examination using these guidelines, laryngeal nerve paresis (as shown by LEMG) exists approximately 86.4% of the time. These guidelines correctly identify which nerve is responsible for paresis identified on examination only 64.3% of the time (unpublished data, Y. Heman-Ackah, MD).

If there is an abnormality in the movement of the cricoarytenoid joint, the vocal fold may be hypomobile or immobile, with evidence of muscular effort. This muscular effort is seen typically as a tensing of the thyroarytenoid muscle during vocal maneuvers without a concomitant change in the position of the vocal fold. When the joint is freely mobile and the muscles are completely paralyzed or nearly totally paralyzed, there is no voluntary movement of the vocal folds on the side that is affected during phonation. However, a jostle sign is seen. The jostle sign is a passive lateral movement of the arytenoid cartilage on the affected side during vocalization that is seen in the region of the muscular process of the arytenoid cartilage. This movement occurs because the mobile arytenoid strikes the arytenoid on the paralyzed side that, in the absence of neuromuscular resistance, is "jostled" laterally by the impact. If the arytenoid is fixed due to dislocation or arthrodesis, this phenomenon will not occur. In addition, paradoxic abduction of the vocal fold may be seen in some patients with unilateral or bilateral RLN paralysis, especially during forceful inspiration. This is due to the Bernoulli effect and is not seen in most patients with mechanical fixation but functioning nerves.

Rigid strobovideolaryngoscopy allows a more magnified and optically superior view of the vibratory function and structure of the vocal fold. Strobovideolaryngoscopy involves the use of synchronized flashing lights through a laryngeal telescope or flexible endoscope to evaluate the function of the mucosal wave of the vocal fold. This procedure is performed usually with a rigid telescope placed through the mouth, usually with the tongue held forward, although strobovideolaryngoscopy can be performed with a flexible laryngoscope. The patient is awake and seated in a forward position during the examination with the chin held slightly upright in a "sniffing" position, which helps to pull the base of the tongue forward so that the larynx can be viewed easily. This magnified view of the vocal folds reveals the presence of structural lesions on the vocal folds that may contribute to the vocal complaint or that may have arisen as a result of the paresis.

ETIOLOGY OF DECREASED VOCAL FOLD MOBILITY

Vocal fold mobility can be affected by disorders of the cricoarytenoid joint, central or peripheral laryngeal neuropathies, or myopathies involving the intrinsic laryngeal muscles. The cricoarytenoid joint can become immobile from inflammatory processes in the joint space, such as those caused by rheumatoid arthritis, gout, other arthritides, trauma, arytenoid dislocation or subluxation during endotracheal intubation, laryngeal fracture, and surgical manipulation in the region of the arytenoid cartilages.[1-9] Because the cricoarytenoid joint is a diarthrodial joint, it can be affected by all disease processes that affect diarthrodial joints elsewhere in the body. Inflammation results in pain, limits joint mobility, and, eventually, causes scarring of the tissues around and within the cricoarytenoid joint, resulting in stenosis and loss of vocal fold mobility. Dysfunction of the muscles of the larynx, as can be caused by amyloidosis, myositis, muscle atrophy, muscular dystrophies, and other myopathies, may affect vocal fold mobility also. Neuromuscular junction disorders such as laryngeal myasthenia may affect the intrinsic muscles of the larynx and limit their mobility. Laryngeal myasthenia is a subset of myasthenia gravis (which is generalized myasthenia throughout the body) and can occur within the context of systemic myasthenia gravis or as an isolated problem without affecting the other muscle systems in the body.[10,11] Laryngeal myasthenia is an autoimmune disorder in which antibodies attack the receptors on the muscle to which acetylcholine binds, destroying the neuromuscular junction. This destruction results in an inability of the muscle to receive signals from the nerve, and the muscle is unable to contract fully in response to neural impulses, resulting in paresis and possibly paralysis of the muscle. Because only those neuromuscular junctions that come in contact with the abnormal antibodies are attacked in myasthenia, some muscles and muscle fibers are not unaffected. This results in variability in the muscle's ability to contract once signaled. In laryngeal myasthenia gravis, typically, this is seen as fluctuations in the ability of the laryngeal muscles to move quickly, resulting in fluctuating asymmetries in vocal fold mobility. Treatment of laryngeal myasthenia is with Mestinon, which inhibits the degradation of acetylcholine at the neuromuscular junction, enhancing neuromuscular transmission.

Amyloidosis is a generalized systemic disorder that can involve the larynx as well as other tissues in the body, most commonly the kidneys.[7,12-16] Amyloidosis is an abnormal accumulation in the tissues of the body of a ground substance, which is amorphous and somewhat like gelatin in the way that it accumulates in the tissues. Accumulation in the larynx adds to the weight of the muscles and inhibits their mobility. Amyloidosis may also accumulate within or around nerve sheaths and cause a peripheral neuropathy of the laryngeal nerves.

Similarly, edema can create a mass effect and result in abnormalities in vocal fold mobility. Edema can result from any form of trauma, such as irradiation, infection, or penetrating and blunt injuries to the neck and larynx.

Myositis is inflammation of the muscle. Inflammatory cells accumulate in the muscle, resulting in tenderness, increased blood flow, increased fluid retention, and increased inflammatory cellular responses. This can occur in response to trauma or infection, but sometimes is idiopathic.[11,17] Like edema and amyloidosis, this chronic inflammation causes a mass effect that inhibits muscle cell mobility. In addition, the inflammation and destruction of the muscle cell membrane or replacement of muscle by abnormal tissue (such as scar) can interfere with the normal transmission of electrical impulses through the muscle, resulting in decreased muscular responses to neural impulses. Similar effects on the laryngeal muscles can be seen with fibromyalgia, scleroderma, lupus, and other autoimmune disorders.

Muscular dystrophies are genetic disorders that are characterized by abnormal muscle metabolism.[18] This abnormal metabolism eventually results in atrophy in many muscles throughout the body, including the larynx.[11] As the muscles in the larynx atrophy, they begin to lose their strength and are no longer able to move as quickly as normal or to produce the same degree of muscle tension, resulting in sluggish and bowed vocal folds. Muscle atrophy of the vocal folds also occurs as a normal part of the aging process and in response to a decline in sex hormone levels, but to a lesser degree than is seen with muscular dystrophies. Acquired myopathies, including dermatomyositis, polymyosits, myoglobinurias, and endocrine myopathies may also limit muscle function and eventually result in muscle atrophy.

Primary neural disorders may also cause decreased vocal fold mobility. Injury to the superior laryngeal nerve and/or the recurrent laryngeal nerve can occur anywhere along their courses from the brainstem to the larynx. Injury to the vagus, superior laryngeal, and/or recurrent laryngeal nerves can be the result of infection, compression, metabolic abnormalities, chronic peripheral neuropathies, or direct injury. Infection results typically from viruses such as herpes simplex, herpes zoster, parainfluenza, influenza, and other viruses that cause the common cold. Infection of the nerves may also result from bacteria such as those that cause syphilis and Lyme disease.[7,19,20] Guillain-Barré is a classic and extreme example of peripheral laryngeal neuropathies that occur as a result of viral infection of the nerves. Compression of the nerve can result from abnormal masses such as lung cancer, carotid aneurysms, aortic aneurysms, metastatic cancer, thyroid tumors, glomus tumors, carotid body tumors, vagal schwannomas, or other tumors of the skull base, neck, mediastinum, or chest. Other processes that may cause a peripheral neuropathy include genetic diseases such as porphyria and Charcot-Marie Tooth disease. Direct injury to the nerve may occur during surgery; during penetrating or blunt trauma to the neck, chest, or skull base; or as a result of endotracheal intubation. Depending upon how much injury is caused, each of these mechanisms can cause paresis or paralysis of the recurrent and/or superior laryngeal nerves.

Processes that affect motor neurons, such as amytrophic lateral sclerosis (ALS), progressive bulbar palsy, spinal muscular atrophy, and poliomyelitis may also affect the laryngeal nerves. Vocal fold paresis and dysphonia may be the initial presenting symptom for all the motor neuron diseases and should always be in the differential diagnosis of vocal fold paresis and paralysis. These disorders typically affect multiple motor nerves, and paresis is usually evident elsewhere, but may be subclinical initially. Fasciculations in the involved muscles are a hallmark of motor neuron diseases and are usually most easily seen in the tongue.

Multiple sclerosis is a demyelinating disorder that can affect both sensory and motor nerves and can be active centrally and/or peripherally. Multiple sensory and motor neuropathies typically occur concommittantly. There may be evidence of demyelination on magnetic resonance imaging of the brain, and lumbar puncture usually reveals elevated mononuclear cells, elevated gamma globulin, and the presence of oligoclonal banding. Symptoms may be rapidly progressive, slowly progressive, or characterized by a series of relapses and remittances.

Both hemorrhagic and ischemic cerebrovascular accidents can result in injury to the motor cortex, internal capsule, and/or brainstem, causing a central paresis or paralysis of the vocal folds. Lesions above the nucleus ambiguus cause contralateral paresis. Those below it cause an ipsilateral paresis.

The etiology of paradoxic vocal fold movements in which the vocal folds appear to inappropriately adduct during inspiration and abduct during expiration remains elusive. With the exception of the paradoxic recruitment patterns seen on LEMG, no other identifiable neurologic abnormality exists in these cases. Because most individuals respond to proton pump inhibitor therapy and laryngeal massage, laryngopharyngeal reflux is thought to play a major role in the pathogenesis of this disorder.

Metabolic abnormalities that can cause disorders in the laryngeal nerves include diabetes mellitus and thyroid abnormalities. These metabolic abnormalities can cause abnormal nerve function that is sometimes reversible, as with thyroid abnormalities alcoholism, thiamine, vitamin B12 deficiencies, and lead poisoning, and sometimes are irreversible, such as with diabetes mellitus.[21] The most common thyroid abnormality associated with reversible paresis is Hashimoto's thyroiditis (unpublished data, Y. Heman-Ackah, MD). Treatment of Hashimoto's thyroiditis with cyclo-oxygenase II (COX-2) inhibitors has been associated with a reversal of the paresis and improvement in the vocal symptoms (unpublished observations,

Y. Heman-Ackah, MD).[22-24] Diabetes mellitus is thought to cause nerve dysfunction via small vessel ischemia of the laryngeal nerves.[11,25] There is some speculation that hypercholesterolemia and hypertriglyceridemia may cause paresis through similar mechanisms. However, substantiating data are lacking.

Compression, infection, and trauma cause nerve dysfunction because they interfere with the transmission of neural impulses. The initial stage of nerve injury results in inhibition of flow of axoplasm, a process termed neuropraxia. With neuropraxia, the nerve remains intact and return of function occurs when the pressure on the nerve from the offending agent is removed. If the offending agent causes excessive pressure on the nerve, demyelination will occur via Wallerian degeneration, and nerve transmission will be compromised. This phase is termed axonotmesis, and full recovery typically occurs with regeneration. After a period of Wallerian degeneration, if the offending agent persists, the endoneural tubules will become injured. Loss of the endoneural tubules effectively removes the "highway" that guides nerve regeneration. In most cases, synkinesis will occur with regeneration. Because each nerve within a nerve sheath contains several hundred nerve fibers, when the regeneration occurs, some of the fibers may misconnect, joining with nerve fibers adjacent to their original ending within the nerve sheath, which leads to a phenomenon called synkinesis. When synkinesis occurs, impulses that the brain tries to send to one muscle are redirected through this misconnection to another muscle. For instance, both the posterior cricoarytenoid muscle and the thyroarytenoid muscle are innervated by the recurrent laryngeal nerve. If the recurrent laryngeal nerve is injured and synkinesis occurs, the posterior cricoarytenoid muscle may be reinnervated by nerve fibers from neurons that originally innervated the thyroarytenoid muscle. Normally, when the brain signals the thyroarytenoid muscle to contract for speech, it signals the posterior cricoarytenoid muscle to relax so that the thyroarytenoid can adduct the vocal folds. In the presence of synkinesis, the signal from the brain to the thyroarytenoid muscle may be rerouted to the posterior cricoarytenoid muscle via this misconnection. As a result, when the person tries to speak, the posterior cricoarytenoid muscles will contract, opening the vocal folds and causing a breathy voice.

If the nerve is severed during surgery or as the result of neck trauma, paralysis of the muscles innervated by the nerve will result. Unless the nerves are surgically reconnected, clinically useful reinnervation is unlikely to occur spontaneously, and permanent paralysis usually will ensue. In general, the absence of innervation results in muscle atrophy and degeneration. If surgical reinnervation is performed, it most likely will result in synkinesis for reasons explained above. Even with synkinesis, the neural input received by the muscle usually is enough for the muscle to maintain its tone and avoid severe atrophy. Functional mobility of the vocal folds is unlikely to occur with surgical innervation procedures or in the face of synkinesis.

SUMMARY

Any process that impairs nerve function, muscle function, or skeletal joint mobility may impair motion of the vocal folds. This chapter has reviewed principles and selected examples of such conditions, but there are many more. The list includes, but is not limited to, benign and malignant tumors of the larynx, other systemic and inflammatory diseases, including granulomatous diseases, and laryngopharyngeal reflux (which can induce inflammatory arthritis and cricoarytenoid arthrodesis). LEMG is helpful in determining the etiology and the severity of vocal fold mobility disorders in a majority of cases of impaired vocal fold mobility, as discussed in the following chapters.

REFERENCES

1. Grossman A, Martin JR, Root HS. Rheumatoid arthritis of the cricoarytenoid joint. *Laryngoscope.* 1961;71:530–544.
2. Polisar IA. The crico-arytenoid joint. a diarthrodial articulation subject to rheumatoid arthritic involvement. *Laryngoscope.* 1959;69:1129–1164.
3. Bridger MW, Jahn AF, van Vostrand AW. Laryngeal rheumatoid arthritis. *Laryngoscope.* 1980;90:296–303.

4. Lawry GV, Finerman ML, Hanafee WN, Mancuso AA, Fan PT, Bluestone R. Laryngeal involvement in rheumatoid arthritis. a clinical, laryngoscopic, and computerized tomographic study. *Arth Rheum.* 1984;27: 873–882.

5. Goodman M, Montgomery W, Minette L. Pathologic findings in gouty cricoarytenoid arthritis. *Arch Otolaryngol.* 1976;102:27–29.

6. Paulsen FP, Jungmann K, Tillmann BN. The cricoarytenoid joint capsule and its relevance to endotracheal intubation. *Anesth Analg.* 2000;90:180–185.

7. Sataloff RT. Common infection and inflammations and other conditions. In: Sataloff RT. *Professional Voice: The Science and Art of Clinical Care.* 3rd ed. San Diego, Calif: Plural Publishing, Inc.; 2005: 807–814.

8. Sataloff RT, Feldman M, Darby KS, Carrol LM, Spiegel JR. Arytenoid dislocation. *J Voice.* 1987;1:368–377.

9. Sataloff RT, Bough ID, Spiegel JR. Arytenoid dislocation: diagnosis and treatment. *Laryngoscope.* 1994;104:1353–1361.

10. Nieman RF, Mountjoy JR, Allen EL. Myasthenia gravis focal to the larynx. Report of a case. *Arch Otolaryngol.* 1975;101:569–570.

11. Sataloff RT, Mandel S, Rosen DC. Neurological disorders affecting the voice in performance. In: Sataloff RT. *Professional Voice: The Science and Art of Clinical Care.* 3rd ed. San Diego, Calif: Plural Publishing, Inc; 2005:847–870.

12. Cohen AS. Amyloidosis. In: Wilson JD, Braunwald E, Isselbacher KJ, Petersdorf RG, Martin JB, Fauci AS, Root RK, eds. *Harrison's Principles of Internal Medicine.* 12th ed. New York, NY: McGraw-Hill Inc; 1991:1417–1421.

13. Hellquist H, Olofsson J, Sokjer H, Odkvist LM. Amyloidosis of the larynx. *Acta Otolaryngol (Stockh).* 1979;88:443–450.

14. Berg AM, Troxler RF, Grillone G, Kasznica J, Kane K, Cohen AS, Skinner M. Localized amyloidosis of the larynx: evidence for light chain composition. *Ann Otol Rhinol Laryngol.* 1993;102:884–889.

15. Bennett JD, Chowdhury CR. Primary amyloidosis of the larynx. *J Laryngol Otol.* 1994;108:339–340.

16. Lewis JE, Olsen KD, Kurtin PJ, Kyle RA. Laryngeal amyloidosis: a clinicopathologic and immunohistochemical review. *Otolaryngol Head Neck Surg.* 1992;106:372–377.

17. Bradley WG, Tandan R. Dermatomyositis and polyomyositis. In: Wilson JD, Braunwald E, Isselbacher KJ, Petersdorf RG, Martin JB, Fauci AS, Root RK, eds. *Harrison's Principles of Internal Medicine.* 12th ed. New York, NY: McGraw-Hill, Inc; 1991;2108–2111.

18. Mendell JR, Griggs RC. Muscular dystrophy. In: Wilson JD, Braunwald E, Isselbacher KJ, Petersdorf RG, Martin JB, Fauci AS, Root RK, eds. *Harrison's Principles of Internal Medicine.* 12th ed. New York, NY: McGraw-Hill Inc; 1991;2112-2114.

19. Rabkin R. Paralysis of the larynx due to central nervous system syphilis. *Eye Ear Nose Throat Monthly.* 1963;42:53.

20. Neuschaefer-Rube C, Haase G, Angerstein W, Kremer B. Einseitige rekurrensparese bei verdacht auf Lyme-borreliose [Unilateral recurrent nerve paralysis in suspected Lyme borreliosis]. *HNO.* 1995;43:188-190.

21. Anderson TD, Anderson DD, Sataloff RT. Endrocrine dysfunction. In: Sataloff RT. *Professional Voice: The Science and Art of Clinical Care.* 3rd ed. San Diego, Calif: Plural Publishing, Inc; 2005:537-550.

22. McComas AJ, Sica RE, McNabb AR, Goldberg WM, Upton AR. Neuropathy in thyrotoxicosis. *N Engl J Med.* 1973;289:219-221.

23. Misiunas A, Niepomniszcze H, Ravera B, Faraj G, Faure E. Peripheral neuropathy in subclinical hypothyroidism. *Thyroid.* 1995;5:283-286.

24. Torres CF, Moxley RT. Hypothyroid neuropathy and myopathy: clinical and electrodiagnostic longitudinal findings. *J Neurol.* 1990;237:271-274.

25. Shuman CR, Weissman B. Recurrent laryngeal nerve involvement as a manifestation of diabetic neuropathy. *Diabetes.* 1968;17:302.

CHAPTER 4

Basic Aspects of the Electrodiagnostic Evaluation

Electromyography (EMG) evaluates the integrity of the motor system by recording action potentials (electrical activity) generated in the muscle fibers.[1-3] EMG is useful particularly for evaluating disorders affecting lower motor neurons, peripheral nerves, neuromuscular junctions, and muscles. EMG should be considered an extension of the physical examination rather than solely a laboratory procedure. Following a thorough and careful examination of the patient, the muscles to be evaluated by EMG are selected prior to beginning the study. Also, abnormalities detected by EMG should be interpreted within the context of the clinical impressions. For those interested, other texts provide a comprehensive presentation of EMG in the diagnosis and treatment of the neurologic disorders,[1-3] and suggestions for further reading may be found in Appendix III.

BASIC NEUROPHYSIOLOGY

The interior of a muscle or nerve cell is electrically negative with respect to its exterior. This electrical potential difference is called the resting membrane potential. In muscles it is on the order of 90 millivolts; for lower motor neurons it is about 70 millivolts. This resting membrane potential reflects the difference in ionic concentration that exists across the cell membrane and the selective permeability of the cell membrane. The intracellular and interstitial fluids are in osmotic and electrical equilibrium with each other; however, the distribution of the ions between the two compartments is unequal. The intracellular compartment has a high concentration of potassium while the extracellular compartment has a high concentration of sodium and chloride. This inequality of ionic concentration is maintained by an active energy-dependent transport mechanism. With the application of an appropriate stimulus, nerves and muscles generate action potentials. The action potential is a fast and transient reversal of the membrane potential caused by a temporary change in membrane permeability. This action potential is propagated along the fiber without decrement. In order to generate the propagating action potential, the membrane must be depolarized to a minimum level known as the membrane threshold potential.[4,5] The motor unit consists of a single lower motor neuron and the muscle fibers that it innervates. Therefore, it includes the cell body of the lower motor neuron in the spinal cord, its axon with its terminal arborization, the neuromuscular junctions, and all the muscle fibers innervated by them (Figure 4–1). The innervation ratio of the muscle is the ratio of the total number of muscle fibers to the total number of motor axons supplying them. The innervation ratio in small muscles such as the laryngeal muscles, external rectus oculi, tensor tympani, and platysma muscles is approximately 25:1 as compared to the innervation ratio of the medial head of the gastrocnemius (a large muscle), which is approximately 1700:1. Muscles with low innervation ratios are typically required to perform finely graded movements. Muscles with high innervation ratios are typically involved in coarser activity. The individual muscle fibers belonging to a given motor unit are scattered diffusely in the muscles without grouping.[6] There are two types of muscle fibers based on histochemical characteristics.

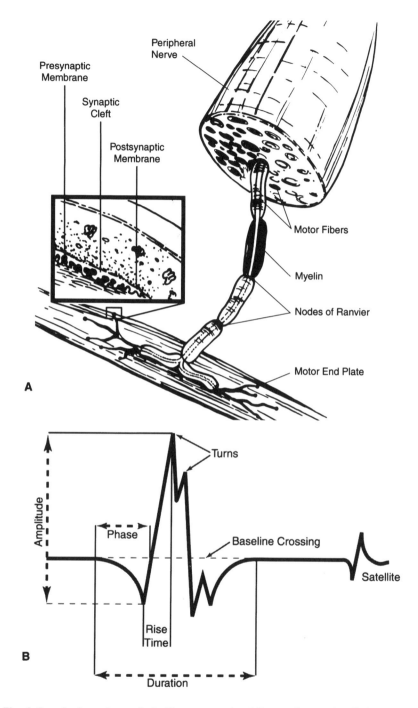

Fig 4-1. **A.** A motor unit. **B.** Components of the action potential generated from a motor unit.

Type 1 fibers are rich in mitochondrial oxidative enzymes but poor in myofibrillar adenosine triphosphatase (ATPase), whereas Type 2 fibers, are rich in myofibrillar ATPase and low in mitochondrial oxidative enzymes (Table 4–1). The muscle fibers of an individual motor unit are all of the same histochemical type. The lower motor neuron has trophic influence on the muscle fiber so that a muscle fiber may change its histochemical characteristics when reinnervated by another motor unit. Type 1 muscle fibers are best suited for producing low-intensity tension for a long time; Type 2 fibers are best suited for generating high tension for a short time.[7] In the spinal cord, smaller motor neurons innervate Type 1 fibers and large motor neurons innervate Type 2 fibers (Table 4–2). Smaller

TABLE 4–1 Properties of Muscle Component of the Motor Unit

Properties	Type S Motor Unit	Type FR Motor Unit	Type FF Motor Unit
Histochemical type	1	2A	2B
Capillary supply	Extensive	Extensive	Sparse
Contractile properties			
—Resistance to fatigue during repetitive stimulation	High	Moderate	Low
—Stimulation rate for fused tetanic contraction	Low	High	High
—Twitch response	Slow	Fast	Fast
—Twitch and tetanus tensions	Small	Moderate	Large
Energy-yielding metabolic pathways	Oxidative	Anaerobic glycolysis +oxidative	Anaerobic glycolysis
Reactivity with histochemical stains for			
—Mitochondrial oxidative enzymes	High	Moderate to High	Low
—Myofibrillar ATPase	Low	High	High
—Phosphorylase	Low	High	High

TABLE 4–2 Properties of Motor Neuron Component of the Motor Unit

Properties	Type S Motor Unit	Type FR Motor Unit	Type FF Motor Unit
Duration of after-hyperpolarization	Long	Short	Long
Firing pattern during activity			
—Firing frequency	About 20 Hz	Up to 100 Hz	Up to 100 Hz
—Firing pattern	Continuous	Bursts	Bursts
Intensity of stimulation required for activation	Low	Moderate	High
Power of accommodation	Low	Moderate	High
Size	Small	Moderately large	Large

motor neurons are typically activated at low muscle tension; therefore, they are the first ones to be observed during the electromyographic evaluation. Large motor neurons are recruited during high muscle tension and are, therefore, seen during maximal muscle contraction. Small motor neurons fire at a lower rate, typically less than 20 Hz; large motor neurons are capable of firing at rates as high as 100 Hz. With aging there is a significant loss of motor neurons in the anterior horn cells. This causes an increase in the innervational ratio of the surviving units.[8]

THE ELECTRODIAGNOSTIC APPARATUS

Bioelectrical potentials from the muscles and/or nerves being examined are detected by an active recording electrode connected to a differential amplifier with a typical common mode rejection ratio of 100,000:1 and a high input impedance of at least 100,000. The frequencies of muscle action potentials range between 2 Hz and 10,000 Hz; and the frequency band of the electromyography machine is typically set at 10 Hz to 10,000 Hz. The reference electrode is also connected to the amplifier. The signal of interest is measured as the potential difference between the active and reference electrodes. The patient must be grounded to reduce the risk of electrical injury and 60 Hz interference. The electrodiagnostic signal is displayed on a cathode ray oscilloscope in real time and can be heard through a loudspeaker. The amplified signal can then be monitored visually and acoustically. The signal can be stored permanently on magnetic tape, a computer disk, or paper. In addition to the qualitative analysis used most commonly, quantitative EMG assessment is also possible. In modern systems, the amplifier signal is also connected to an analog-to-digital converter, a microprocessor, and a video monitor for a digital display of the signal. This permits rapid mathematical manipulation of the raw data. In addition, there is an electrical stimulator incorporated into the system that is connected to the microprocessor and the oscilloscope so that it can trigger the recording system when stimulation is provided. The ability of an amplifier to reject common mode signals is indicated by its common mode rejection ratio (CMRR). The higher the ratio, the greater the ability of the amplifier to reject common mode potentials. In clinical electromyography, amplifiers with a CMRR of 10,000 are preferred, which means that unequal potential differences between the two inputs of the amplifier will be amplified 10,000 times more than potentials equal to both inputs.[9,10] In most EMG laboratories, sophisticated, multichannel systems are utilized. There are several excellent systems available commercially. They have many advantages, including permitting simultaneous, multichannel recording; but EMG systems are fairly expensive. For otolaryngologists who plan to utilize laryngeal electromyography for needle guidance when injecting botulinum toxin or for occasional diagnostic purposes, less expensive, conveniently portable systems are now available such as the device manufactured by Xomed (Jacksonville, Fla) (Figure 4-2). In its basic form, this EMG unit provides only auditory information and single-channel recording; but it can be connected to a computer to provide a visual display. Such compact devices are also valuable for bedside, in-patient testing of patients with laryngeal trauma to help differentiate between arytenoid injury and vocal fold paralysis; they are especially convenient during evenings and weekends, when formal EMG laboratory facilities may not be available. Another cost-effec-

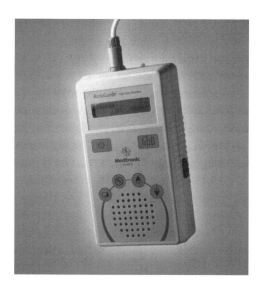

Fig 4–2. Portable, cost-effective, single-channel EMG device (Medtronics-Xomed, Jacksonville, Fla).

tive option for otolaryngologists is the use of the brainstem-evoked response (ABR) audiometer found in many offices. Most ABR units can be used (sometimes with minor modifications) for at least single-channel EMG recordings. However, although such devices can be used for specific clinical indications when formal EMG cannot be performed, they should be utilized in addition to, not in place of, a sophisticated, multichannel EMG system for diagnostic testing. The flow of current in biological tissues occurs as a result of the movement of ions. In electronic systems, it is due to the movement of electrons. The conversion of ionic activity into electron movements occurs at the electrode-tissue interface. Electrodes usually are made of a metal that is a good conductor of electricity. Surface and needle electrodes are used in electromyography. Surface electrodes are placed on the skin or mucosa and do not penetrate the surface. Although they are noninvasive, they are the least selective electrode type. Surface electrodes are used in the study of nerve conduction velocity and neuromuscular transmission. The potential that is recorded represents the sum of all individual potentials produced by the nerve or muscle fibers that are activated. These electrodes are not suitable for recording details of electrical events associated with individual motor units. Typically, surface electrodes consist of a metal disk with a diameter of 0.5 to 2.5 cm. There are several types of needle electrodes: monopolar, bipolar, concentric, hooked-wire, and single-fiber (Figure 4–3A). The monopolar needle electrode is a solid stainless steel needle that is insulated except at its tip. The recording area from this electrode is circular. Therefore, potentials tend to be larger and longer, and have more phases than those recorded with concentric needle electrodes. This is because

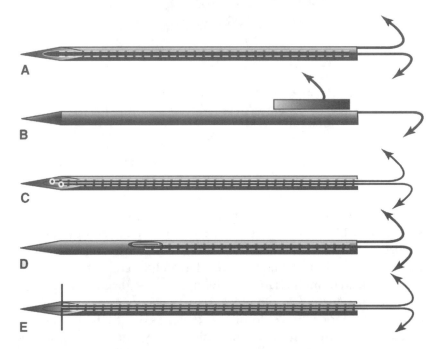

Fig 4–3. A. Needle electrodes. **(A)** is a concentric electrode with the active electrode embedded in the bevel of the needle. The needle shaft serves as the reference. **(B)** is a monopolar electrode with the active electrode occupying the needle tip. The reference electrode may be a surface electrode placed on the skin or a needle electrode placed elsewhere. **(C)** is a bipolar electrode with 2 platinum wires and a grounded outer shaft. **(D)** is a single-fiber electrode. The reference is the cut end of a wire embedded in a hole in the side of the shaft. **(E)** is two hooked-wire electrodes inside an insertion needle. *(continues)*

more muscle fibers are within the zone of detection, and there is less cancellation due to potentials being recorded from the cannula of the electrode (Figure 4-3B). The reference electrode is at a remote location on the body and may be a surface electrode.

The concentric needle electrode consists of a hollow steel needle with a silver, steel, or platinum wire that runs through the needle, which is insulated fully except at the tip. The potential difference between the outer shaft of the needle and the tip of the wire is measured by connecting it to one side of the differential amplifier. Because the electrode cannula acts as a shield, the electrode has directional recording characteristics controlled by the angle and position of the bevel. Therefore, simple rotation of the electrode may alter significantly which individual motor units are recorded. The bipolar electrode is a hollow needle containing two platinum wires, each of which is insulated except at its tip. The outer shaft is grounded and the two internal wires are each connected to one side of the differential amplifier so that the potential difference between the two wires is measured. The recording range of the bipolar electrode is restricted to the area between the two wires within the shaft which makes it unsatisfactory for many

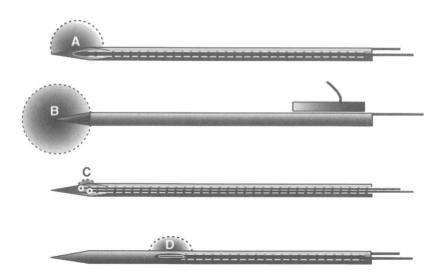

Fig 4-3. *(continued)* **B.** Zones of detection for concentric **(A)**, monopolar **(B)**, bipolar **(C)**, and single-fiber **(D)** needle electrodes.

routine clinical purposes. The potentials are shorter and lower in voltage than those recorded with concentric needle electrodes.[11] For single-fiber EMG, a fine wire that is capable of recording a single muscle fiber action potential is embedded at the tip of a needle shaft that acts as the reference. A hooked-wire electrode is completely insulated except at the tip, which is hooked. A needle is used to insert the electrode. When the needle is withdrawn, the hook on the end of the wire acts as a barb, stabilizing the position of the electrode in the muscle. Obviously, these electrodes cannot be repositioned once they have been placed, but they bend easily and can thus be withdrawn without difficulty. Hooked-wire electrodes are extremely well tolerated and can be left in place for long periods of time (hours, or even days).

SAFETY CONSIDERATIONS

Current may leak from the electrodiagnostic system due to capacity coupling. This current leakage may lead to death or injury in a patient by causing ventricular fibrillation. To minimize the risk of this complication, every patient must be grounded. Also, the current leakage from the instrument should not exceed 10 microamperes.[12]

BASIC COMPONENTS OF EMG EXAMINATION

Basic components of electromyographic examination are discussed in this chapter partially, and in more detail in Chapter 5. An EMG examination is performed and evaluated in consists of four parts: (1) during insertion, (2) at rest, (3) during minimal voluntary contraction, and (4) during maximal voluntary contraction. Characteristics of laryngeal EMG during minimal and maximal voluntary contraction arc discussed in Chapter 5.

Insertional Activity

Insertional activity is the electrical signal that is produced as the needle is introduced into the muscle. Normally, insertion of the needle causes bursts of electrical activity. These should last no more than several hundred milliseconds. This burst of electrical activity results from the fact that the needle itself has some electrical energy that, when placed near the muscle membrane, causes a relative change in the surrounding electrical energy. If the electrical charges surrounding the muscle membrane are unstable, such as occurs during early nerve and muscle injuries, the insertional activity will be prolonged. With late nerve and muscle injuries, healing sometimes results in replacement of normal muscle with scar tissue or fat, which insulates the remaining muscle fibers and causes a decrease in the insertional activity.

Spontaneous Activity

Spontaneous activity refers to the presence of electrical activity in the muscle when it is at rest in a resting muscle. Under normal conditions, there should be no spontaneous electrical activity usually at rest. Electrical activity arises from neural impulses that signal the muscle to contract. Spontaneous electrical activity occurs in a severely denervated muscle with unstable electrical charges. The presence of spontaneous activity implies that the muscle is degenerating and/or that the nerve has been injured and that the process that caused the injury is ongoing. This is true in muscles throughout the body, including those in the larynx.[13,14] Spontaneous activity usually begins 2 to 3 weeks after denervation has occurred because it takes a while for the nerve to degenerate to a degree that results in the absence of electrical impulses from the nerve to the muscle. This degree of denervation occurs only with severe nerve injury, and the presence of spontaneous activity indicates a poor prognosis for recovery. Once regeneration begins, the muscle begins to receive electrical impulses from the regenerating nerve and the spontaneous activity ceases.

Waveform Morphology

Waveform morphology refers to the shape, amplitude, and duration of the motor unit potentials, which are the electrical signals captured by EMG. The normal laryngeal motor unit potential is biphasic; that is, it has an upward positive spike and a downward negative spike. It also has an amplitude of 200 to 500 microvolts and a duration of about 5 to 6 milliseconds. The amplitude of the motor unit potential reflects the number and the strength of the muscle fibers innervated by one nerve ending. The duration of the motor unit potential reflects the velocity of the neural input, which is influenced by the insulation of the nerve. Nerves that are insulated well and have an intact and functioning sheath are able to transmit electrical impulses faster than those that are not, as electrical impulses are then transmitted from one node of Ranvier to another. The shape of the motor unit potential reflects changes in the electrical activity of the muscle membrane. Under normal circumstances, this is biphasic. The waveform morphology of the motor unit potential provides information regarding likelihood of recovery. After injury, the nerve goes through a process of denervation followed by regeneration. The length of time that denervation and regeneration occur can vary from one situation to another and can last for periods of weeks to months each. It is unknown what determines how much a nerve will denervate or regenerate. During denervation, there is no neural input into the muscle, and, thus, no abnormal waveforms are produced. Abnormal motor unit potential morphologies are produced during the period of regeneration. During the early phases of regeneration, tiny nerves begin to course back into the muscles that have atrophied during the period of time that they were denervated. Early in regrowth, the insulation of the nerve is decreased. The combination of the tiny, minimally insulated nerves and the weak muscle fibers produces electrical signals on LEMG that are seen as motor unit potentials that have small amplitudes, long durations, and polyphasic shapes. These waveforms are sometimes referred to as nascent units; they imply the presence of a recent nerve injury. As the regeneration progresses, the nerves become healthier and better insulated through regrowth of their sheaths; the muscle fibers become stronger and gain more mass. Not all of the nerve fibers regenerate. Fibers that do regenerate usually branch more extensively than they did before the injury, and they spread to innervate as many denervated muscle fibers as possible. The motor unit potentials that are produced as a result of this ongoing regeneration have greater amplitudes than normal, are polyphasic, and have a prolonged duration. These motor unit potentials are usually described as being polyphasic or as giant polyphasic potentials; their presence implies an old nerve injury.

If the nerve is uninjured and the muscle is damaged, the morphology of the motor unit potential is different. The nerve is intact and functioning well, so the duration of the motor unit potential is normal. The electrical charges in the muscle membrane are abnormal, resulting in a polyphasic shape. The amplitude, which reflects the decreased muscle mass and force of contraction, is decreased.

Recruitment

Recruitment refers to the serial activation of motor units during increased voluntary muscle contraction. Normally, as the intensity of the muscle contraction increases, the motor units have increased activity and new motor units are "recruited" to maintain the strength of the contraction. This is seen on LEMG as an increase in the number and density of motor unit potentials. This density of motor unit potentials is the recruitment. Thus, recruitment reflects the degree of innervation, which is a reflection of the number of active nerve fibers within a given muscle.

COMMON ABNORMAL EMG FINDINGS

Increased insertional activity occurs when the burst of electrical potential produced by insertion or movement of the needle electrode in the muscle lasts more than several hundred milliseconds. This is an indication of muscle membrane instability and occurs in both myopathic and neurogenic processes. Insertional activity also can be reduced, indicating loss of muscle fiber and replacement of it by fibrotic tissue or lipoid degeneration. This is observed in end-stage myopathic and some neuropathic processes.

At rest, different kinds of abnormal spontaneous activity can be observed. *Fibrillation potentials* (Figure 4–4) are spontaneous, single-fiber muscle action potentials with a typical amplitude of several hundred microvolts and durations of less than 2 milliseconds, firing regularly at 1 to 50 Hz. They can occur spontaneously or with

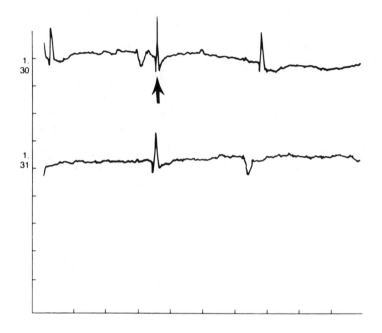

Fig 4-4. Fibrillation potentials *(solid arrow)* and positive sharp wave recorded from the right thyroarytenoid muscle in a patient with recurrent laryngeal neuropathy.

movement of the needle. They typically have a biphasic or triphasic appearance with an initial positive deflection. This abnormality is seen more commonly when denervation has occurred. Rarely, it can be seen in myopathic processes as well. A *positive sharp wave* is characterized by a large positive deflection of several hundred microvolts lasting less than 2 milliseconds, followed by a negative deflection of 10 to 30 milliseconds and regular firing at 1 to 50 Hz. Fibrillation potentials and positive sharp waves usually occur together and produce very characteristic noises on the loudspeaker that some describe as sounding like "machine gun firing," thus, allowing one to identify these potentials even without looking at the oscilloscope screen. It takes approximately 2 to 3 weeks after denervation occurs to observe fibrillation potentials or positive sharp waves. After a nerve injury, the presence of fibrillations and positive sharp waves indicates denervation and axonal loss.

Complex repetitive discharges (Figure 4-5) occur when a group of muscle fibers discharges repetitively in near synchrony through *ephaptic* activation. These discharges typically have an abrupt onset and cessation and a bizarre configuration. The discharge rate is anywhere between 5 and 100 Hz, with an amplitude of 100 μV to 1 mV. This abnormality indicates chronicity, and it can be observed in both neuropathic and myopathic processes. *Myotonic potentials* (Figure 4-6) are repetitive discharges at rates of 20 to 150 Hz and amplitudes of 20 μV to 1 mV, with the appearance of fibrillation potentials or positive sharp waves. The amplitude and the frequency of the potentials wax and wane, which causes a characteristic "dive bomber" sound in the loudspeaker of the EMG machine. These potentials occur spontaneously with insertion of the needle, with percussion of the muscle, or with voluntary contractions. They are indicative of muscle membrane instability and are observed most

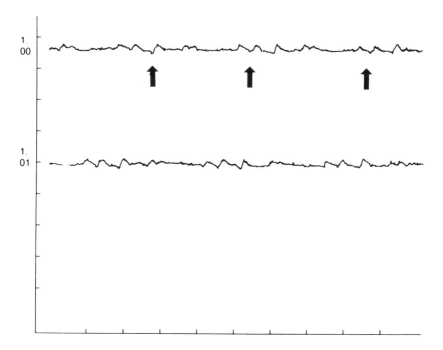

Fig 4–5. Low amplitude complex repetitive discharges *(arrows)* recorded from the right thyroarytenoid muscle in a patient with recurrent laryngeal neuropathy.

MYOTONIC DISCHARGE

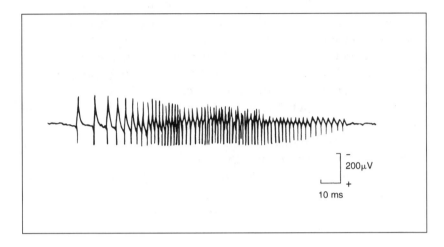

Fig 4-6. Myotonic potentials.

commonly in disorders of clinical myotonia, such as myotonic dystrophy. Rarely, they can be observed in chronic neurogenic and myopathic processes such as fibromyalgia without clinical myotonia.

During minimal voluntary muscle contraction, the morphology of the motor unit potential is evaluated. Abnormalities are characterized by changes in the duration, amplitude, and number of phases (Figure 4-7). In a neuropathic process, the motor unit potential typically has a prolonged duration and increased number (more than 4) of phases (Figure 4-8). During early reinnervation, the amplitude is decreased and, when reinnervation is completed, the amplitude is increased. In myopathic processes, the duration of the motor unit potential is short, with an increased number of phases and decreased amplitude. With maximal muscle contraction, the interference pattern and recruitment are evaluated. When a nerve impulse arrives at a motor end plate, muscle fibers depolarize and contract. Because there are numerous fibers in any muscle motor unit, and their distances from the neuromuscular junction vary, not all muscle fibers in a motor unit contract simultaneously. In fact, laryngeal muscles generally exhibit polyphasic contraction.[15,16] In reality, numerous motor units are involved during muscle contraction. As the contraction increases, motor units fire more frequently and,

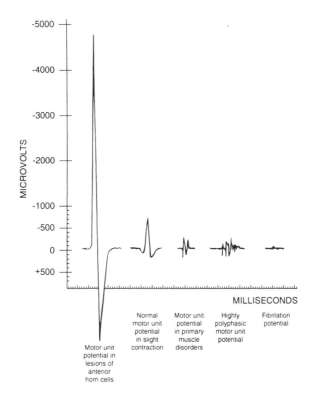

Fig 4-7. Differences in the appearance of the motor unit potential in diseases.

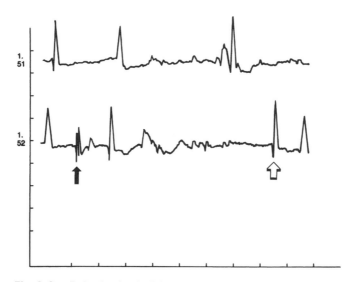

Fig 4-8. Polyphasic *(solid arrow)* and normal *(open arrow)* motor units recorded from the left cricothyroid muscle.

progressively, additional motor units are activated. Consequently, recorded motor units overlap, creating an interference pattern. Potentials that can be identified visually and audibly during very weak contraction overlap during stronger contraction; therefore, some fading can result in a recruitment pattern in which some of the spikes appear to be lost. By looking at, or listening to, the EMG signal, a skilled electromyographer can determine the condition of the muscle. For example, under normal circumstances, the interference pattern described above is present. In complete paralysis, initially there is electrical silence; however, positive sharp waves or fibrillation potentials generally appear within a few weeks. Reinnervation is characterized by larger motor units with polyphasic, high-amplitude, and long-duration responses. There is usually loss of motor units following paralysis, which results in decreased recruitment (a less dense interference pattern). In neuropathic processes, there is decreased recruitment, with a few motor units firing at high frequency and a decreased interference pattern (Figure 4-9). In a

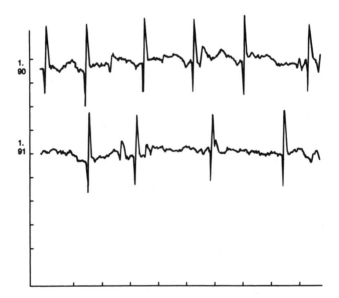

Fig 4-9. Incomplete interference pattern showing decreased recruitment with rapid discharge rate recorded from the right thyroarytenoid muscle in a patient with recurrent laryngeal neuropathy.

myopathic process, there is rapid and early recruitment with a low voltage, and a full interference pattern in the context of a weak muscle contraction.

SINGLE-FIBER EMG

Single-fiber EMG evaluates individual muscle fibers. The technique was introduced in 1963 by Ekstedt and Stalberg.[17] It can be helpful in patients with neuromuscular junction abnormalities such as myasthenia gravis,[18-21] and those with denervating disorders such as amyotrophic lateral sclerosis (ALS). The needle electrode recording surface is located along the shaft (Figure 4–3). A wire 25 μm in diameter is embedded in a small resin port 7.5 mm from the tip,[22] with the electrode shaft acting as the reference. Because of the small recording surface, it is possible to record selectively from the isopotential lines generated by a single muscle fiber action potential.[22-24] The electrode must be placed extremely close to the fiber of interest. Visual and acoustical information is used to adjust placement of the electrode for optimal recording. Movements of as little as 100 μm alter the amplitude of the potential substantially.[24,25] The low-pass filter (high frequency) is set at 8 to 10 kHz, and the high-pass filter (low frequency) is set at about 500 Hz to filter out interference from nearby muscle fibers. A delay line on the display monitor with a threshold trigger is required to display single muscle fiber action potentials during successive discharges. Sweep speeds of 2 or 5 msec per division are utilized. Single muscle fiber action potentials are normally only a few milliseconds in duration. Recordings are made generally during uniform voluntary contraction of moderate intensity. Recordings can be made from a single fiber, or from two muscle fibers innervated by the same motor unit. Typically, two fibers from the same motor unit (a potential pair) are recorded to allow measurements of jitter and fiber density. The double potential is located by auditory feedback that has been compared to the sound of castanets.[22] Peak-to-peak amplitude should be greater than 200 μV, and spike rise time should be less than 300 μsec (usually between 67 and 200 μsec, with a median of 112 μsec).[24] The waveform should be stable during successive discharges.[26] The spike duration usually ranges from 265 to 800 μsec (with a median of 470 μsec) and voltage ranges from 0.7 to 25.2 mV (with a median of 5.6 mV).[26]

Jitter measures the difference between two time-locked firing potentials of the same motor unit, specifically the variability of their interpotential interval (IPI) during successive discharges.[22,27] Recordings do not have to be made at maximum amplitude but must record at least 50 stable, successive discharges from a potential pair. The IPI is a reflection of the length of the distal axon branch from the motor axon to the end plate, conduction velocity along the distal axon branch, neuromuscular transmission, distance from the recording electrode to the end plate, and muscle fiber conduction velocity.[24] The most important factors are conduction velocity along the distal axon branch, neuromuscular transmission, and muscle fiber conduction velocity. Variation in neuromuscular transmission is dominant if the IPI is 1 msec or less and the firing rate is uniform.[22] Variation in conduction velocity along the distal axon branch and variation in muscle fiber conduction velocity may be dominant factors if the IPI is 10 msec or longer and the discharge rate is not uniform.[22] Thus, to obtain the necessary information about neuromuscular transmissions it is preferable to record jitter with IPIs of 4 msec or less.[22] Jitter is expressed as the mean value of consecutive differences (MCD) in the IPIs, measured over short periods of time. In normal subjects, jitter is usually 10 to 50 μsec (MCD), but it is occasionally as low as 5 μsec (MCD).[28] In patients with myasthenia gravis, jitter may exceed 100 msec (MCD). In myasthenia, impulse blocking may occur, which is a failure of one or more of the time-locked single muscle fiber action potentials to fire in the triggered discharge.[22] Bimodal jitter occurs when variability is distributed around two separate means. This occurs in 1 out of 20 jitter measurements in normal muscles[24] and may be a source of error if it is not recognized and analyzed appropriately. The interested reader is referred to other literature for additional details regarding the complex techniques of jitter measurement and calculation.[22,28-37]

Fiber density provides an index of the number of muscle fibers that comprise a motor unit.[22,38,39] Four or five measurements are made in at least four sites within the muscle, and 20 different single muscle fiber action potentials at different sites within the muscle are typically measured. Measurements are made during maximal amplitude. The recording radius of a single-fiber electrode is approximately 300 μm.[22] The optimized potential and all the other time-locked potentials that belong to the same motor unit that can be recorded during the discharge of the motor unit potential are counted. The total number of single-fiber muscle action potentials recorded at these 20 different sites are added together, then divided by 20 to determine the mean fiber density.[22,40] Sixty to seventy percent of the time in most muscles, fiber density measurements record only a single muscle fiber action potential,[40] because 76% of all muscle fibers belonging to a motor unit are separated from other muscle fibers from that motor unit.[41] These characteristics (percentage of fibers separated from other fibers in a motor unit; fiber density) have not been studied in specific laryngeal muscles. During fiber density recording, it is also possible to determine the mean of the interspike intervals (MISI). This is determined by dividing the total duration of the potentials that are time-locked to the triggered potential by the number of intervals within the potential complex.[22] The MISI is typically increased in myopathies, such as polio and muscular dystrophies, and in early reinnervation. Single-fiber EMG is more sensitive than conventional repetitive stimulation studies and is felt to be abnormal in 99% of patients with generalized myasthenia gravis. However, studies on patients with focal myasthenia (such as ocular myasthenia and, particularly, laryngeal myasthenia) are probably less definitive. In individuals with localized myasthenia, the percentage of patients with neuromuscular junction abnormalities in whom the condition is confirmed by single-fiber EMG may not be as high as it is when the condition involves forearm muscles, but the technique may still be superior to other conventional EMG techniques and repetitive studies. Single-fiber EMG may be particularly helpful in patients with neuromuscular junction problems such as myasthenia gravis, but it can be influenced by drugs such as pyridostigmine bromide (Mestinon, ICN Pharmaceuticals) and can also show abnormalities in any disorder in which there is a failure of neuromuscular junction transmission, including neuropathies and myopathies. Individuals with ALS and those with nerve injury can produce similar abnormalities on single-fiber EMG. Therefore, the technique cannot be used alone in the absence of clinical data and other EMG studies to establish a definitive diagnosis.

Jitter measurements can be very helpful in patients with suspected myasthenia, and fiber density can be helpful in individuals with denervation, both recent and long-standing, but there are pitfalls. Single-fiber EMG should be interpreted in the context of the clinical presentation and results of other electrodiagnostic procedures.

REFERENCES

1. Daube JR. AAEM minimonograph #11: needle examination in clinical electromyography. *Muscle Nerve.* 1991;14:685–700.
2. Kimura J. *Electrodiagnosis in Diseases of Nerve and Muscles: Principles and Practice.* 2nd ed. Philadelphia, Pa: FA Davis Company; 1989.
3. Lindestad P. *Electromyographic and Laryngoscopic Studies of Normal and Disturbed Voice Function.* Stockholm, Sweden: Departments of Logopedics and Phoniatrics and Clinical Neurophysiology. Huddinge University Hospital; 1994.
4. Kandel ER, Schwartz JH, Hessell TM. Ion channels. In: *Principles of Neuroscience.* 4th ed. New York, NY: McGraw-Hill; 2000:105–125.
5. Kandel ER, Schwartz JH, Hessell TM. Propagated signaling: the action potential. In: *Principles of Neuroscience.* 4th ed. New York, NY: McGraw Hill; 2000:150–175.
6. Burke RE. Physiology of motor unit. In: Engle AG, Franzini-Armstrong, C, eds. *Myology.* New York, NY: McGraw-Hill; 1994:464.
7. Dubowit CV, Pearse AGE. A comparative histochemical study of oxidative enzyme and phosphorylase activity in skeletal muscles. *Histochemie.* 1960;2:105–117.
8. Aminoff MJ. Properties and functional organization of motor units. In: Aminoff MJ. *Electromyography in Clinical Practice.* 3rd ed. New York, NY: Churchill Livingston; 1998:33.
9. Gitter AG, Stolov WG. Instrumentation and measurement in electrodiagnostic medicine, part I. *Muscle Nerve.* 1995;18:799–811.
10. Gitter AG, Stolov WG. Instrumentation and measurement in electrodiagnostic medicine, part II. *Muscle Nerve.* 1995;18:812–824.
11. Guld C, Rosenfalck A, Willison RG. Report of the committee on EMG instrumentation: technical factors in recording electrical activity of muscles and nerve in men. *Electroencephalogr Clin Neurophysiol.* 1970;28:399–413.
12. Starmer CF, McIntosh HD, Whalen RE. Electrical hazards and cardiovascular function. *N Engl J Med.* 1971;284:181–186.

13. Koufman JA, Walker FO. Laryngeal electromyography in clinical practice: indications, techniques, and interpretation. *Phonoscope.* 1998;1: 57-70.

14. Sittel C, Stennert E, Thumfort WF, Dapunt U, Eckel HE. Prognostic value of laryngeal electromyography in vocal fold paralysis. *Arch Otolaryngol Head Neck Surg.* 2001;127:155-160.

15. Faaborg-Andersen, K. Electromyographic investigation of intrinsic laryngeal muscles in humans. *Acta Physiol Scand.* 1957;41(suppl 140): 1-149.

16. Haglund S. The normal electromyogram in human cricothyroid muscle. *Acta Otolaryngol (Stockh).* 1973;75:478-453.

17. Ekstedt J, Stalberg E. A method of recording extracellular action potentials of single muscle fibres and measuring their propagation velocity in voluntarily activated human muscle. *Bull Am Assoc EMG Electrodiagn.* 1963;10:16.

18. Ekstedt J, Stalberg E. Single muscle fibre electomyography in myasthenia gravis. In: Kunze, K, Desmedt JE, eds. *Studies in Neuromuscular Disease.* Basel, Switzerland: Karger; 1975:157-161.

19. Howard JF, Sanders DB. Serial single-fiber EMG studies in myasthenic patients treated with corticosteroids and plasma exchange therapy. *Muscle Nerve.* 1981;4:254.

20. Schwartz MS, Stalberg E. Myasthenia gravis with features of the myasthenic syndrome: an investigation with electrophysiologic methods including single fibre electromyography. *Neurology.* 1975;25:80-84.

21. Stalberg E, Ekstedt J, Broman A. The electromyographic jitter in normal human muscles. *Electroencephalogr Clin Neurophysiol.* 1975;31: 429-438.

22. Stalberg E, Trontelj JV. *Single Fiber Electromyography in Healthy and Diseased Muscle.* 2nd ed. New York, NY: Raven Press; 1994.

23. Ekstedt J, Stalberg E. How the size of the needle electrode leading-off surface influences the shape of the single muscle fibre action potential in electromyography. *Comput Programs Biomed.* 1973;3:204-212.

24. Ekstedt J, Stalberg E. Single fibre electromyography for the study of the microphysiology of the human muscle. In: Desmedt JE, ed. *New Developments in Electromyography and Clinical Neurophysiology.* Basel, Switzerland: Karger; 1973:89-112.

25. Fuglsang-Frederiksen A, LoMonaco M, Dahl K. Electrical muscle activity during a gradual increase in force in patients with neuromuscular diseases. *Electroencephalogr Clin Neurophysiol.* 1984;57:320-329.

26. Ekstedt J. Human single muscle fibre action potentials. *Acta Physiol Scand.* 1964;61(suppl 226):1-96.

27. Stalberg E, Ekstedt J, Broman A. The electromyographic jitter in normal human muscles. *Electroencephalogr Clin Neurophysiol.* 1971; 31(5):429-438.

28. Ekstedt J, Stalberg E. Abnormal connections between skeletal muscle fibers. *Electroencephalogr Clin Neurophysiol.* 1969;27:607-609.

29. Thiele B, Stalberg E. The bimodal jitter: a single fibre electromyographic finding. *J Neurol Neurosurg Psychiatry.*1974;37:403-411.

30. Stalberg E. Propagation velocity in human single muscle fibers in situ. *Acta Physiol Scand.* 1966;70(suppl 287):1-112.

31. Mihelin M, Trontelj JV, Stalberg E. Muscle fiber recovery functions studied in the double pulse stimulation. *Muscle Nerve.* 1991;14: 739-747.

32. Sanders DB, Stalberg EV. AAEM minimonograph #36: single-fiber electromyography. *Muscle Nerve.* 1996;19:1069-1083.

33. Ekstedt J, Nilsson G, Stalberg E. Calculation of the electromyographic jitter. *J Neurol Neurosurg Psychiatry.* 1974;37:526-539.

34. Stalberg E, Ekstedt J, Broman A. The electromyographic jitter in normal human muscles. *Electroencephalogr Clin Neurophysiol.* 1971; 31(5):426-438.

35. Bromberg MB, Scott DM, Ad Hoc Committee of the AAEM Special Interest Group Single Fiber EMG. Single fiber EMG reference values: reformatted in tabular form. *Muscle Nerve.*1994;17(7):820-821.

36. Gilchrist JM, Ad Hoc Committee of the AAEM Special Interest Group on Single Fiber EMG. Single fiber EMG reference values: a collaborative effort. *Muscle Nerve.* 1992;15:151-161.

37. Hilton-Brown P, Stalberg E. The motor unit in muscular dystrophy, a single fibre EMG and scanning EMG study. *J Neurol Neurosurg Psychiatry.* 1983;46:981-995.

38. Gath I, Stalberg E. On the measurement of fibre density in human muscles. *Electroencephalogr Clin Neurophysiol.* 1982;54:699-706.

39. Trontelj JV. H-reflex of single motoneurones in man. *Nature.* 1968; 220:1043-1044.

40. Stalberg E, Thiele B. Motor unit fibre density in the extensor digitorum communis muscle: single fibre electromyographic study in normal subjects of different ages. *J Neurol Neurosurg Psychiatry.* 1975;38: 874-880.

41. Brandstater ME, Lambert EH. Motor unit anatomy, type and spatial arrangement of muscle fibers. In: Desmedt JE, ed. *New Developments in Electromyographyand Clinical Neurophysiology.* Basel, Switzerland: Karger; 1973:14-22.

CHAPTER 5

Laryngeal Electromyography

Laryngeal electromyography (LEMG) was introduced in 1944 by Weddel et al[1] and was advanced substantially in the 1950s by Faaborg-Andersen and others.[2-4] Additional research by various investigators in the 1960s and 1970s began to clarify the potential importance of EMG in laryngology.[5-29] Throughout the 1980s and 1990s, laryngeal electromyography evolved into an invaluable adjunct to laryngo-logic assessment, diagnosis, and treatment of voice disorders.[30-34] Laryngeal EMG is easy to perform, is well-tolerated in the office setting, and presents minimal risks to patients. It is useful in the evaluation of numerous laryngeal disorders, allowing clinicians to differentiate among upper motor neuron, lower motor neuron, peripheral nerve, neuromuscular junction, myopathic, and mechan-ical disorders. It is also useful in establishing prognosis in laryngeal nerve palsies and for guidance during the injection of botulinum toxin in spasmodic dysphonia. A skilled laryngeal electromyographer is an immeasurable asset to the voice care team. Laryngeal EMG evaluates the integrity and integrative function of the laryngeal motor system. It is best regarded not as a laboratory test, but rather as an extension of the laryngologic examination. Judgments regarding when to use laryngeal EMG, selection of the muscles to be studied, and the choice of EMG techniques depend upon a comprehensive history and physical examination. In addition, laryngeal EMG requires expert interpretation, taking the clinical scenario into account. Electromyography is usually performed by a neurologist, physiatrist, electrophysiologist, or laryngologist skilled in this procedure.

There are few contraindications to laryngeal electromyography. It is relatively contraindicated in patients with coagulopathy or those taking anticoagulant medications such as warfarin; but it can be performed even in patients with bleeding tendencies when the clinical value of the electrophysiologic information justifies the slightly increased risk. The authors have performed laryngeal EMG on numerous occasions for patients taking anticoagulants, without complications thus far. Repetitive stimulation studies should not be performed on patients who have pacemakers.

TECHNICAL ASPECTS OF LARYNGEAL ELECTROMYOGRAPHY

The physiologic basis and general principles of EMG have been discussed previously and will not be reviewed here. This chapter instead emphasizes technical considerations important specifically to EMG of laryngeal muscles. The selection of electrode type for laryngeal EMG remains controversial and should be guided by the clinical indications for the study. Surface electrodes placed on the skin or mucosa are not invasive, but they are the least specific and least sensitive. Because the laryngeal muscles are small and in close proximity to each other, surface electrodes are generally not useful for diagnostic EMG. However, they still have some value for the laryngologist. Endotracheal tubes with built-in surface electrodes are utilized to monitor recurrent laryngeal nerve function during neck operations such as thyroid surgery,[34] for example. Surface electrodes have also been used to record posterior cricoarytenoid muscle activity and other laryngeal muscle function[35,36] and for biofeedback.[37,38] Invasive concentric or monopolar needle electrodes are used most commonly for laryngeal testing. A concentric electrode consists of a needle that serves as a reference electrode and a central insulated core. The tip is beveled, and the area of sampling is controlled by the angle of the bevel. Concentric electrodes are used frequently because of their consistent, reproducible results.[39-42] However, slight changes in position or angulation can alter results. Near threshold levels of activity, concentric electrodes many even be capable of recording single motor units. Monopolar electrodes are needle electrodes that are insulated except for a small distance near their tips; the reference electrode is placed at a remote location and may be a surface electrode. Monopolar electrodes are not as selective as concentric needle electrodes. Thus, concentric electrodes are preferable when one is interested in identifying single motor unit potentials or selectively sampling activity that is very close to the electrode. This can also be accomplished with small bipolar needle electrodes that contain two insulated wires within the needle cannula. However, monopolar needle electrodes may provide a more useful analysis of the overall activity of an intrinsic laryngeal muscle. Some investigators feel that monopolar electrodes are inaccurate because they may detect unwanted signals from adjacent laryngeal muscles. Usually, however, this is not a problem. Because of their ease of use monopolar electrodes provide faster assessment of overall recruitment response of a given intrinsic laryngeal muscle. Much of the other information sought (presence of fibrillation potentials or sharp waves, for example) can be detected reliably with monopolar electrodes as well and this is suitable for most clinical purposes. Detailed information about individual motor units is best obtained using connecting electrodes or hooked-wire electrodes. In addition, monopolar electrodes can be constructed of hollow needles that can be used for therapy. Therapeutic needle electrodes are used for EMG-guided injection of substances such as botulinum toxin. Single-fiber EMG may be valuable in confirming the diagnosis of conditions such as myasthenia gravis and postpolio syndrome. Traditionally, hooked-wire electrodes have been used in laryngeal study, primarily for research, but they may have clinical value as well. Hooked-wire electrodes are flexible, generally remain in good position despite patient movement, and are well tolerated over time. Therefore, they may be valuable for studying laryngeal function during phonatory tasks and swallowing, and in numerous positions of the neck. They may also be placed in children under general anesthesia and then used for laryngeal electromyography during performance of phonatory tasks when the child has awakened. Hooked-wire electrodes are fine wires (30 gauge) that are insulated completely except at the tip, which is hooked. A needle is used to insert hooked-wire electrodes. When the needle is withdrawn, the hooks on the heads of the wires act as barbs, stabilizing electrode position in the muscle. The electrodes cannot be repositioned, but they can be withdrawn easily because they bend. Their flexibility and small size make them extremely well-tolerated. Since Basmajian and Steco reported the concept of hooked-wire electrodes in 1962,[43] they have been used for a variety of purposes. Despite early recognition of their advantages for long-term study of a dynamic system, like the larynx,[16] they have not gained widespread popularity for routine clinical use. Nevertheless, some clinicians use hooked-wire electrodes to study the posterior cricoarytenoid muscles, using an inserter designed by W. Thumfart and marketed by the Wolf Company (Vernon Hill, Ill); Dr. Peak Woo uses custom-made wire electrode arrays consisting of up to four electrodes in clinical practice (Peak Woo, MD, personal communication, 2000). Hooked-wire electrodes may have technical disadvantages. Muscle contraction may alter responses by changing the distance between the two electrodes with regard to the muscle fibers they are intended to measure, and with regard to each other.[23] The authors use percutaneous monopolar needle electrodes routinely. The patient is placed in the supine position, with the neck extended. Because the procedure is generally not very painful, and because local anesthesia may alter results (especially in the cricothyroid muscle), local anesthesia is not used. A surface electrode is used for the ground electrode, and a reference (also surface) is placed on the cheek. For diagnostic purposes, routinely we test cricothyroid, thyroarytenoid, and posterior cricoarytenoid muscles. In some cases, additional muscles are tested as well. If there are questions regarding hysteria, malingering, or synkinesis, simultaneous recordings of abductors and adductors are obtained. In cases of laryngeal dystonia, electrical recordings may be coordinated with acoustical data. Blitzer et al observed that the normal delay between the onset of the electrical signal and the onset of the acoustic signal (0–200 milliseconds) can be increased to a delay of 500 milliseconds to 1 second in patients with spasmodic dysphonia.[40,44] After cleaning the skin with alcohol, the needle electrode is inserted into the muscle belly. The cricothyroid (CT) notch is the anatomic reference for needle insertion. To locate the CT notch, the patient's neck is extended and the cricoid cartilage is identified. Immediately above the cricoid cartilage is a small depression, which is the CT notch, also known as the CT space, and the CT membrane region. The CT notch may be difficult to find in obese patients or those who have had a tracheotomy. The CT muscles are evaluated by inserting the needle approximately 0.5 cm from the midline and angled laterally 30 to 45 degrees (Figures 5-1 and 5-2). The needle first passes through the sternohyoid muscle. The CT muscle is approximately 1 cm deep. To validate the position of the electrode, the patient is asked to phonate /i/ at a low pitch and then asked to raise the pitch. If the electrode is in a normal CT muscle, the EMG activity will increase sharply. To evaluate the thyroarytenoid (TA) muscle, the needle is inserted approximately 0.5 cm from the midline of the CT notch and is angled superiorly 30 to 45 degrees. The TA muscle is encountered approximately 1 to 2 cm beneath the skin. If the patient coughs, that generally indicates that the needle has penetrated the airway and is causing irritation of the mucosa. In that case, the needle should be withdrawn and reinserted. The position of the needle is validated by asking the patient to say /i/. During this maneuver, there will be a sharp and sustained increase in EMG activity. If the needle is in the lateral cricoarytenoid muscle (LCA) there will be an increase and rapid drop-off in EMG activity. The posterior cricoarytenoid muscle (PCA) can be accessed by rotating the larynx and passing the electrode posterior to the thyroid lamina, or by passing a needle through the cricothyroid membrane, airway, and cricoid cartilage posteriorly. The latter technique is successful usually only in nonossified larynges, such as those of young women. The PCA lies lower in the neck than many physicians realize; inserting the electrode too high is a common reason for difficulty in locating the PCA. Position is confirmed through detection of increased EMG activity during sniffing, and with much less EMG activity during swallowing and phonating the sound /i/.

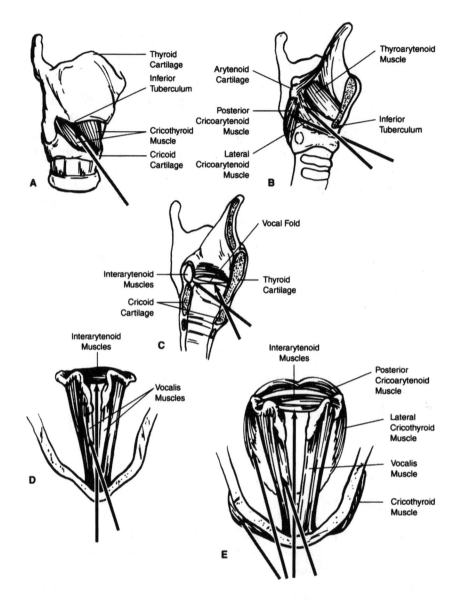

Fig 5-1. Position of insertion of electrodes into the laryngeal muscles for electromyography. Muscles illustrated include the cricothyroid **(A)**, lateral and posterior cricoarytenoid muscles **(B)**, and the interarytenoid and thyroarytenoid (vocalis) muscles (vocal fold) **(C)**. Also shown are the positions of insertion into five major laryngeal muscles **(D, E)**: (1) CT, (2) LCA, (3) PCA, (4) TA, (5) IA. Numbers correspond to the needle position for insertion into the respective muscles. It is possible in some patients to place a needle in the PCA by passing through the 1A (E,5) and the cricoid cartilage (usually a few mm to the left or right of the midline posteriorly).

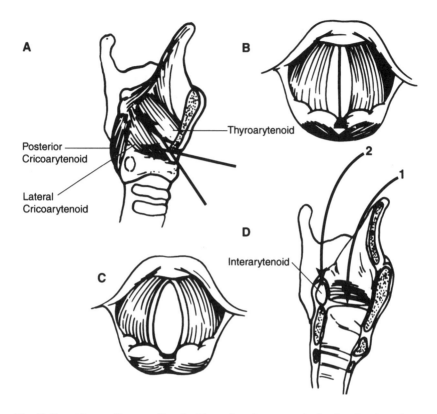

Fig 5-2. Alternative method of inserting laryngeal electrodes for electromyography, including a modified approach to the vocalis (thyroarytenoid) muscles **(A)**, peroral point of insertion into the posterior cricoarytenoid muscles **(B)**, peroral point of insertion into the interarytenoid muscles **(C)**, and peroral point of insertion into the thyroarytenoid **(D1)** and interarytenoid **(D2)** muscles.

The lateral cricoarytenoid muscle (LCA) is slightly lower, more lateral, and more posterior than the TA. Successful insertion can be confirmed electrically because of a difference in the firing pattern between the TA and LCA. When the patient is asked to say /i/ with an electrode in the TA, there is a fairly constant level of activity throughout phonation. In the LCA, a large spike of activity is seen as the LCA brings the vocal process toward the midline, but activity drops promptly to a lower level as it is maintained in the adducted position.

Thyroarytenoid, posterior cricoarytenoid, lateral cricoarytenoid, and interarytenoid electrodes can also be positioned indirectly under flexible fiberoptic guidance or directly in the operating room.[45,46] As with EMG elsewhere in the body, laryngeal EMG examination consists of four parts, including insertion, rest, minimal voluntary contraction, and maximal voluntary contraction. With insertion of the needle into the muscle or with any movement of the needle, bursts of electrical activity are produced by the mechanical stimulation of the muscle membrane. They last no more than several hundred milliseconds (Figure 5-3). At rest, no electrical activity is recorded, but laryngeal muscles are rarely at physiologic rest. When the electrode is in close proximity to the neuromuscular junction, normal physiologic activity, endplate spikes, and noise can be recorded. With minimal voluntary contraction, 1 or 2 motor unit potentials can be recorded with a firing rate of 2 to 5 per second. The average duration of the motor unit potentials recorded from laryngeal muscles is 3 to 7 milliseconds with an amplitude of 150 to 800 μV.[3,10,17,24] Most of the studies used to determine these parameters utilized concentric electrodes. Using monopolar elec-

INSERTION ACTIVITY

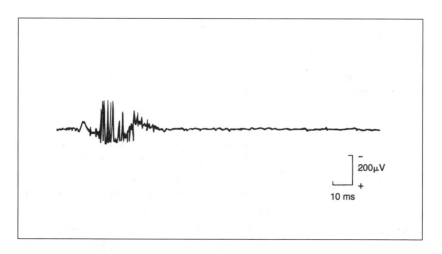

200μV

10 ms

Fig 5-3. Normal insertional activity.

trodes, findings of 5 to 6 milliseconds with an amplitude of 200 to 500 μV may be more typical[47] (Figure 5-4). As the intensity of the contraction increases, the firing rate of the motor unit potentials increases and new and larger motor units are recruited, filling the oscilloscope screen so that single motor unit potentials cannot be distinguished from each other. This is known as a *full interference pattern*[48] (Figure 5-5), and it is generally achieved at about 30% of maximal isometric contraction.[42] If a concentric electrode is used, only approximately 100 to 150 fibers are within recording distance of the electrode tip; during full muscle effort, motor units fire asynchronously at frequencies of 30 to 50 motor units per second. So, the potentials generated occur at intervals of about 1 millisecond.[49]

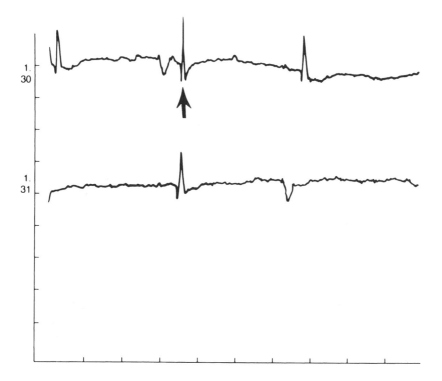

Fig 5-4. Normal motor unit (*arrow*) recorded from the cricothyroid muscle.

RECRUITMENT PATTERN

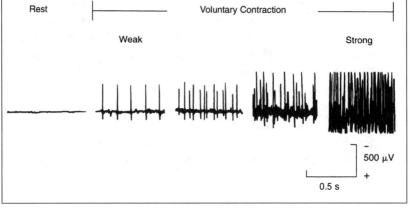

Fig 5-5. Normal recruitment pattern.

Interpretation of Laryngeal EMG

Laryngeal EMG may be evaluated qualitatively or quantitatively, to some extent. The importance of the skill of the electromyographer and the subjective judgments implicit in EMG interpretation must be understood. Qualitative assessment is performed by listening to the amplified signal and by viewing the oscilloscope display. A skilled electromyographer can tell much about the condition of the neuromuscular complex. It is important to remember that single motor unit action potentials of laryngeal muscles normally have slight polyphasia (1 to 3 phases), so this should not be interpreted as abnormal.[3,10] However, the presence of greater than four phases in laryngeal muscles should be considered abnormal. The electrical silence associated with complete denervation is interpreted easily, so long as the electromyographer is certain that the needle is in the appropriate muscle. Other abnormalities such as fibrillation potentials, positive sharp waves, giant motor units, and abnormal amplitudes and durations are also recognized readily. The somewhat thinned interference pattern associated with the loss of motor units following reinnervation may be more difficult to recognize if the electromyographer does not have extensive experience with laryngeal muscles. The electromyographer using auditory and visual data, together with his or her knowledge of anticipated maximal muscle activity, can estimate the percentage of normal recruitment response in each laryngeal muscle tested with excellent consistency, according to our experience (Figure 5-6). This has proven useful clinically. More formal quantitative analysis of laryngeal EMG signals has proven challenging. Several investigators have used integrated, digitally smoothed signals.[9,26,50,51] This method utilizes firing frequency and averaged amplitude of the signal. The amplitude of the signal data is reported as a percentage of the estimated maximal electrical activity of the muscle. This is similar to the percentage recruitment method used clinically, and discussed above. However, approximation of maximal muscle activity in the larynx may be as challenging in the laboratory as it is in clinical practice, and results must be considered approximate at best. In addition, this method of digitally smoothing and integrating signals loses data with regard to the relationship between firing frequency and amplitude.

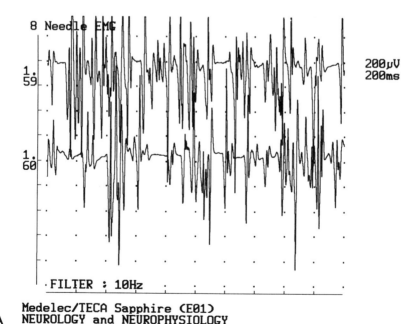

Fig 5-6. **A.** Full recruitment pattern at maximal contraction. *(continues)*

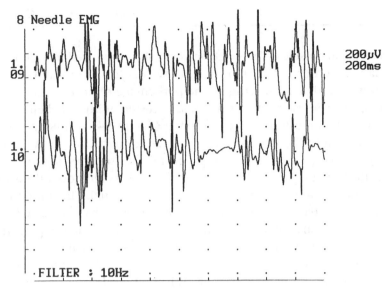

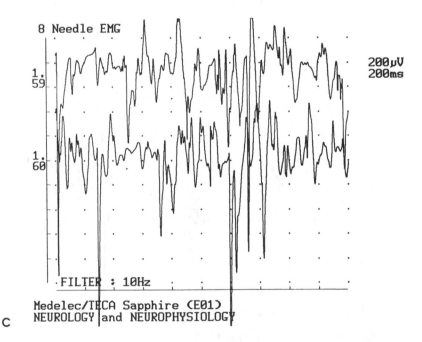

Fig 5-6. *(continued)* **B.** Maximal contraction, motor unit recruitment decreased approximately 30%. **C.** Maximal contraction, motor unit recruitment decreased approximately 50%. *(continues)*

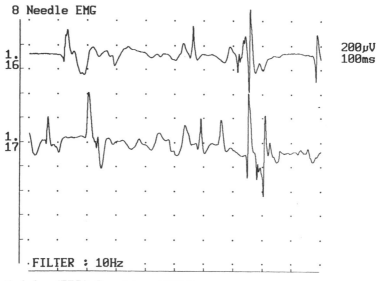

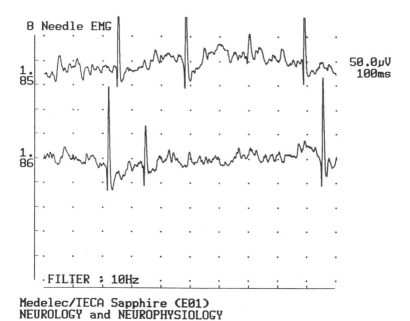

Fig 5-6. *(continued)* **D.** Maximal contraction, motor unit recruitment decreased approximately 70%. **E.** Maximal contraction, motor unit recruitment decreased approximately 80 to 90%.*(continues)*

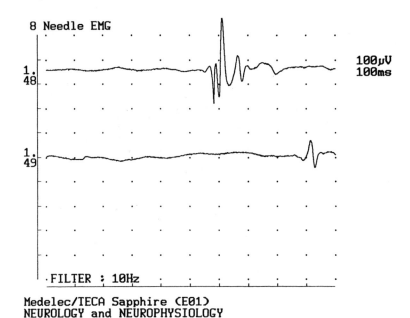

Medelec/TECA Sapphire (E01)
F   NEUROLOGY and NEUROPHYSIOLOGY

Fig 5-6. *(continued)* **F.** Maximal contraction, revealing a single poly-phasic motor unit potential. Approximately one year following recurrent laryngeal nerve injury. Essentially 100% reduced recruitment.

Investigators have also attempted to quantify electrical muscle activity by measuring the amplitude of the signal, ignoring its frequency or density.[3,18,29] It should be noted that amplitude can be affected by many factors including age and temperature,[41] as well as distance of the needle electrode from the muscle fibers being tested. The rise time, or distance between the first negative deflection and its subsequent peak, is related to this distance and should be less than 200 microseconds for assessment of a motor unit potential to be meaningful.[40,41] Because of the basic principles of neurophysiology, direct comparison of EMG muscle recordings from examination to examination is not valid. This is especially true when small areas are sampled through use of concentric bipolar or hooked-wire electrodes, but the task appears less problematic clinically when larger areas are sampled using monopolar electrodes. However, concentric electrodes also permit turns/amplitude analysis of the interference pattern, permitting assessment of some of the motor units that "disappear." This technique was introduced in 1964[52] and requires computer analysis. A "turn" is two successive shifts in amplitude of 100 μV or more. Mean amplitude between turns over time is measured. Mean amplitude is greatest during maximal muscle contraction effort, but the number of turns is greatest at about 50% of maximal effort[53,54] with increasing force. Small muscles show a greater increase in turns and a smaller increase in amplitude than large muscles[55]; females have lower values for turns and amplitude than males. Electrical recordings from several positions within a muscle are used to create a "scattergram" for quantitative turns/amplitude analysis. Turns/amplitude analysis has been used in larger skeletal muscles in both normal and pathologic conditions, and has been found helpful in discriminating electrical differences comparing normal muscles to those in patients with peripheral nerve lesions[52,55-58] and in neurogenic disorders.[58] Fuglsang-Frederiksen and coworkers have demonstrated that turns/amplitude analysis is most effective when the muscle is contracting at about 30% maximal force.[58-60] Nevertheless, there is very little experience using this technique for laryngeal muscles, and there is evidence to suggest that turns/amplitude analysis may not be as sensitive as visual analysis or other methods of analyzing motor unit potentials.[61,62] The most definitive investigation of turns/amplitude analysis of laryngeal EMG was carried out by Lindestad, who found that it was less valuable than conventional analysis for diagnostic purposes.[49]

CLINICAL APPLICATIONS OF LARYNGEAL EMG

Laryngeal EMG can be useful in the diagnosis of a variety of disorders affecting the laryngeal muscles or their innervation. Some of the most common situations in which laryngeal EMG can be helpful include:

1. Lower motor neuron disorders

2. Evaluation of recurrent or superior laryngeal nerve palsy/ paralysis

3. Prognosis for recovery of vocal fold paralysis

4. Differentiation of paralysis from cricoanytenoid joint fixation

5. Malingering and psychogenic dysphonia

6. Basal ganglia disorder

7. Laryngeal dystonias and tremors

8. Myopathic disorders

9. Neuromuscular junction disorders

10. Upper motor neuron disorders

Lower Motor Neuron and Laryngeal Nerve Disorders

In early lower motor neuron (LMN) and laryngeal nerve disorders, there is increased insertional activity. Positive sharp wave and fibrillation potentials are frequently observed. Complex repetitive discharges and, rarely, myotonic discharges may also occur. The motor unit potential is prolonged, with an increased number of phases, and the amplitude can be either increased or decreased. There is an incomplete interference pattern, with decreased recruitment and rapid firing of the remaining motor units. Laryngeal EMG can be useful for the evaluation of hoarseness and dysphagia in patients with LMN problems such as amyotrophic lateral sclerosis, Guillain-Barré, polio, postpolio syndrome,[63-65] multiple system atrophy (Parkinson's Plus syndrome),[66,67] Charcot-Marie-Tooth disease[68] and other anterior horn cell, nerve root, and peripheral nerve degenerative diseases, and post-traumatic disorders. The laryngeal EMG abnormalities are much the same as those described for laryngeal nerve disorders, as it is a LMN abnormality. Palmer et al[69] found the motor unit action potential recruitment to be the most sensitive (82%) and specific (92%) predictor of lower and upper neuron disorders. In a study of vocal fold paresis, decreased recruitment was found to be present 92.8% of the time (Y. Heman-Ackah and A. Barr, unpublished data).

Laryngeal EMG helps in the evaluation of vocal fold palsy.[70] Simpson et al[71] studied 34 patients with idiopathic vocal fold paralysis confirmed by laryngoscopy and laryngeal EMG. In 29 vocal folds, there was evidence of active and chronic denervation in the

TA muscle, indicating recurrent laryngeal neuropathy. In five cases there was denervation of the CT muscle, indicating superior laryngeal neuropathy. In one case, there was denervation in both the TA and CT muscles, indicating a proximal laryngeal or vagus nerve neuropathy. Koufman et al[72] reported recently on 50 patients with a diagnosis of vocal fold paresis, with dysphonia as the uniform presenting sign. They found that 40% had a combination recurrent laryngeal nerve (RLN) and superior laryngeal nerve (SLN) paresis, 44% had an isolated RLN paresis, and 16% had isolated SLN neuropathy. The clinical importance of superior laryngeal nerve paresis is becoming more widely recognized.[66,67,71,73-76] Laryngeal electromyography is particularly helpful in confirming this diagnosis,[75] which may be responsible for vocal fold bowing, loss of projection, and other difficulties with voice control and endurance. Unrecognized superior laryngeal nerve paresis may also lead to compensatory muscular tension dysphonia that may cause structural pathology such as nodules, pseudocysts, and cysts. In such cases, laryngeal EMG may be invaluable in helping to recognize the underlying primary problem (paresis) and in designing an appropriate therapeutic program. Laryngeal EMG can assist in predicting the recovery of laryngeal paralysis, and studies show a positive predictive value as high as 90%.[73,77-81] The presence of normal motor unit waveform morphology and recruitment (indicating incomplete nerve injury) predicts good functional recovery. Poor functional recovery may be predicted by the presence of positive sharp waves and fibrillations, and by the absence of motor unit potentials (polyphasic or normal).[73,77] However, it should be stressed that the presence of reinnervation does not necessarily guarantee return of function. Synkinesis has been recognized in the larynx at least since 1963.[82] It is possible for opposing muscles to be innervated nearly equally, leaving a reinnervated larynx without appropriate motion. This important problem was studied electromyographically by Blitzer et al.[83] One of the authors (RTS) and Drs. Rontal and Rontal (Michael Rontal, MD, and Eugene Rontal, MD, personal communication, 1997) have utilized botulinum toxin in such situations. Although it may seem counterintuitive to inject botulinum toxin into a "paralyzed" vocal fold, it is possible to use this toxin to eliminate synkinetic reinnervation and improve adduction or abduction (depending on which muscle is injected), as required by the patient's condition. Synkinesis must be distinguished from hysteria and malingering, which also can cause simultaneous firing of abductors and adductors, but in a pattern different from that seen with synkinesis and usually fairly symmetrically bilaterally. Laryngeal EMG also has been found useful in the evaluation of vocal fold paralysis in children, a population somewhat difficult to assess accurately by laryngoscopy and prone to bilateral vocal fold paresis.[84-86]

Laryngeal EMG can be useful in the differentiation of mechanical abnormalities such as vocal fold fixation or arytenoid subluxation from neurologic etiologies by demonstrating normal EMG activity in vocal fold fixation and arytenoids subluxation.[87-90] Sataloff et al[90] and Yin et al[91] have noted EMG abnormalities in some patients with arytenoid dislocation. In the authors' experiences, this is most common in the thyroarytenoid muscle and may be due to direct trauma and/or hemorrhage associated with the injury that caused the dislocation. However, dislocation and paresis can coexist. More than one muscle innervated by the recurrent laryngeal nerve should be tested (including the PCA); a quantitative assessment of laryngeal function is helpful. For example, 30% reduced recruitment response in the thyroarytenoid muscle is abnormal, but it is not sufficient to explain an immobile vocal fold. If all other muscles innervated by the recurrent nerve are normal and the arytenoid is subluxed or dislocated, the EMG abnormality is probably due to post-traumatic muscle injury and scar, and the patient should not be diagnosed with paresis. If there is decreased function in all muscles innervated by the recurrent nerve, then paresis can be diagnosed appropriately even in the presence of an arytenoid dislocation.

Intraoperative laryngeal electrophysiological monitoring during thyroid and laryngotracheal surgery has proven invaluable.[92] The introduction of the Xomed (Jacksonville, Fla) endotracheal tube with RLN sensors provides a convenient method for detecting impending nerve injury during thyroid and other neck surgery, and for avoiding permanent injury.[93] It has advantages (such as ease of placement by a nonlaryngologist) in comparison with needle electrodes, but both techniques may be useful for intraoperative monitoring. It should be noted that thyroid surgery represents the etiology of only 9% of cases of unilateral vocal fold paralysis[94] and that SLN injury not detected currently by intraoperative EMG may be more common in this surgery.[75]

Basal Ganglia Disorders

The insertional activity is normal in basal ganglia disorders. Abnormal spontaneous activity is absent. At rest there may be excessive motor unit potentials, indicating failure of complete relaxation of the muscle. There may also be poor coordination between agonistic and antagonistic muscles, or inappropriate activation. In addition, rhythmic and periodic discharges of motor unit potentials can be observed in patients with voice tremor.[95] Stuttering may also be associated with tremor-like EMG activity.[96]

Dystonia

In laryngeal dystonia, there are intermittent sudden increases in muscle activity coinciding with momentary voice rest.[97-99] The EMG can be helpful in differentiating adductor versus abductor dystonia.[100] Rodriguez et al[101] found abnormal activity in 81.3% of spasmodic dysphonia (SD) patients but found no EMG abnormality predictive of severity. Laryngeal EMG is used routinely to guide botulinum injection in patients with laryngeal dystonia.[102,103] As noted above, an abnormal delay between the onset of electrical and acoustic activity can help confirm a diagnosis of dystonia. EMG may also help identify the muscle(s) affected most by the dystonia, thereby guiding therapeutic intervention.

Myopathic Disorders

The insertional activity in patients with myopathic disorders is either increased or decreased. Some necrotizing myopathies, such as myositis, and some muscular dystrophies can demonstrate positive waves and fibrillations. Complex repetitive discharges and myotonic potentials can occur. The motor unit potential is short, with an increased number of phases anddecreased amplitude. Recruitment is rapid and early, with a full interfer-ence pattern that is of low amplitude. In myotonic dystrophy, myotonic discharges of TA and CT muscles can produce hoarseness.

Neuromuscular Junction Disorders

In myasthenia gravis (MG) and chemical-induced cholinesterase inhibition such as that caused by exposure to insecticides, the insertional activity is normal. There is no abnormal spontaneous activity. With minimal muscle contraction, the motor unit potential exhibits variation in amplitude and duration, reflecting intermittent failure of conduction across the neuromuscular junction. The recruitment and interference patterns are normal. Repetitive nerve stimulation studies are usually abnormal and reveal a lack of increased recruitment with each repetitive stimulation. Myasthenia gravis can be a cause of intermittent and fluctuating hoarseness and voice fatigue. Laryngeal manifestations may be the first and only sign of systemic myasthenia gravis.[104] Laryngeal MG may occur with systemic MG or as a focal disorder similar to ocular MG.

If there is evidence of fluctuating nerve weakness on laryngeal examination, repetitive stimulation studies and edrophonium (Tensilon, Baxter Health Care) testing may be performed. Repetitive stimulation involves presenting the nerve with a series of electrical shocks and recording the neuromuscular response by EMG. The nerve stimulated is often the spinal accessory nerve, which innervates the trapezius muscle. This nerve is chosen because it lies just beneath the skin of the neck and is easy to locate for stimulation. Repetitive stimulation provides information regarding the integrity of the neuromuscular junction. With a normal neuromuscular system, recruitment remains normal during repetitive stimulation. If the stimulation causes a progressively decreasing recruitment response, then an abnormality in the neuromuscular junction is suspected. A decrease in the recruitment response implies that motor units that were previously recruited are unable to be actively and continually recruited during repetitive stimulation. The fact that they were able to be recruited initially and give normal waveform morphology implies that the nerve fibers themselves are intact and that the muscles are able to respond to an impulse signal. The fact that the motor units are unable to keep up with the repetitive stimulation implies that there is an abnormality in the transfer of information across the neuromuscular junction, which is only apparent when the system is stressed. If the laryngeal evaluation is abnormal, or if there are other abnormalities noted during the laryngeal

EMG, then Tensilon testing may be performed. Repetitive stimulation testing is contraindicated in patients with pacemakers.

Tensilon is a drug that inhibits the degradation of acetylcholine in the neuromuscular junction, resulting in increased exposure of the muscle receptors to acetylcholine during neural stimulation. In normal muscles, this has very little effect on muscle activity. In muscles with decreased numbers of available receptors for acetylcholine (as occurs with myasthenia), in those with increased activity of acetylcholinesterase, or in those with decreased release of acetylcholine from the nerve ending, the presence of Tensilon results in increased muscle contraction from the prolonged exposure to acetylcholine. When laryngeal EMG is repeated following administration of Tensilon, the recruitment patterns revert to a more normal pattern with voluntary contraction and with repetitive stimulation. Voice quality may also improve with resolution of breathiness, softness, and fatigue. This positive response to Tensilon further isolates the problem to the neuromuscular junction.

Tensilon testing involves the intravenous injection of edrophonium into a vein and repeating the laryngeal EMG. A syringe containing 10 mg of Tensilon is used for intravenous injection. Initially, 2 mg are injected over 15 to 30 seconds. If there is no reaction after 45 seconds, the remaining 8 mg are injected. If a cholinergic reaction occurs after injection of 2 mg, the test is discontinued and 0.4 to 0.5 mg of atropine sulfate are administered intravenously. Typical signs of cholinergic reaction include skeletal muscle fasciculations, increased muscle weakness, and muscarinic side effects. In patients who have had such reactions, the test may be repeated one-half hour after administration of atropine sulfate. In patients with inaccessible veins, Tensilon may be given as an intramuscular injection. Tensilon testing can also be performed in children, with doses adjusted according to the child's weight.

Tensilon testing is contraindicated in patients with urinary or intestinal obstructions, or in those with known hypersensitivity to anticholinesterase agents. Tensilon is an anticholinesterase drug that inhibits cholinesterase at sites of cholinergic transmissions within 30 to 60 seconds after injection; its effect lasts an average of approximately 10 minutes. Occasionally severe cholinergic reactions occur. Caution must be exercised, particularly in patients with bronchial asthma or cardiac arrhythmias. The transient bradycardia that sometimes occurs following Tensilon injection can be relieved by atropine sulfate, but isolated incidents of cardiac and respiratory arrest have occurred following administration of Tensilon. A syringe containing 1 mg of atropine sulfate should be available at all times for emergency rescue. Tensilon also contains sodium sulfite. Allergic reactions to sulfites can occur and are more common in asthmatic patients than in others. The safety of Tensilon for use during pregnancy or lactation has not be established. Use of Tensilon in pregnant women and nursing mothers is relatively contraindicated.

Upper Motor Neuron Disorders

In upper motor neuron disorders, the insertional activity is normal. There is no abnormal spontaneous activity. The amplitude and duration of the motor unit potential are normal, and there are no excessive polyphasic motor units. Recruitment is decreased. The firing rate of the motor unit is slow. Most upper motor neuron diseases demonstrate hyperactive reflexes with increased tone and no muscle atrophy. There is a paucity of studies in the literature evaluating laryngeal function with EMG in patients with upper motor neuron disorders.

Other Uses

As the use of laryngeal EMG becomes more common, additional clinical and research applications continue to be developed. Its use in the evaluation and treatment of dysphagia also continues to advance.[105,106] New understandings of the interaction between respiration and TA/CT firing may provide additional information regarding the physiology of sudden infant death syndrome (SIDS) and obstructive sleep apnea (OSA), and may advance the development of laryngeal pacing.[107-112]

SUMMARY

Laryngeal EMG is easy to perform and well tolerated in the office setting. It is associated with minimal risks. It is useful in the evaluation of numerous laryngeal disorders, allowing clinicians to differentiate among upper motor neuron, lower motor neuron, peripheral nerve, neuromuscular junction, myopathic, and mechanical disorders. It is also useful in establishing prognosis in laryngeal nerve palsies and for guidance during the injection of botulinum toxin in spasmodic dysphonia. Our experience is similar to that of Koufman et al, who reported 415 laryngeal EMG studies, 83% of which revealed a neuropathic process.[113] They reported unexpected findings in 26% and laryngeal EMG altered clinical management in 40% of cases, highlighting the importance of this simple, quick procedure in the practice of laryngology. We concur and believe that collaboration between the laryngologist and a skilled laryngeal electromyographer is an invaluable and essential asset to the voice care team. However, it should be noted also that there is a striking paucity of evidence-based research to confirm or refute scientifically and incontrovertibly the value of laryngeal EMG for most of the purposes for which we use and recommend it.[114] Additional prospective, controlled laryngeal EMG research should be encouraged and supported, and should be used to formulate formal practice guidelines for clinical use of laryngeal electromyography.

REFERENCES

1. Weddel G, Feinstein B, Pattle RE. The electrical activity of voluntary muscle in man under normal and pathological conditions. *Brain.* 1944;67:178–187.
2. Faaborg-Andersen K, Buchtal F. Action potentials from internal laryngeal muscles during phonation. *Nature.* 1956;177:340–341.
3. Faaborg-Andersen K. Electromyographic investigation of intrinsic laryngeal muscles in humans. *Acta Physiol.* 1957;41 (suppl 140): 1–149.
4. Buchtal F. Electromyography of intrinsic laryngeal muscles. *J Exp Physiol.* 1959;44:137–148.
5. Dedo HH, Hall WN. Electrodes in laryngeal electromyography: reliability comparison. *Ann Otol Rhinol Laryngol.* 1969;78:172–180.
6. Dedo HH. The paralyzed larynx: an electromyographical study in dogs and humans. *Laryngoscope.* 1970;80:1445–1517.
7. English ET, Blevins CE. Motor units of laryngeal muscles. *Arch Otolaryngol.* 1969;89:778–784.

8. Fex S. Judging the movements of vocal cords in larynx paralysis. *Acta Otolaryngol (Stockh).* 1970;263:82–83.

9. Gay T, Hirose H, Strome M, Sawashima M. Electromyography of the intrinsic laryngeal muscles during phonation. *Ann Otolaryngol.* 1972;81:401–409.

10. Haglund S. *Electromyography in the Diagnosis of Laryngeal Motor Disorders* [dissertation]. Stockholm, Sweden: Karolinska Institute, Departments of Otolaryngology and Clinical Neurophysiology; 1973.

11. Haglund S. The normal electromyogram in human cricothyroid muscle. *Acta Otolaryngol (Stockh).* 1973;75:478–483.

12. Haglund S, Knutsson E, Martensson A. An electromyographic study of the vocal and cricothyroid muscles in functional dysphonia. *Acta Otolaryngol (Stockh).* 1974;77:140–149.

13. Hast MH. Mechanical properties of the cricothyroid muscle. *Laryngoscope.* 1966;75:537–548.

14. Hast MH. Mechanical properties of the vocal fold muscles. *Practica Oto-Rhino-Laryngologica.* 1967;33:209–214.

15. Hast MH, Golbus S. Physiology of the lateral cricoarytenoid muscles. *Practica Oto-Rhino-Laryngologica (Basel).* 1971;33:209–214.

16. Hirano M, Ohala J. Use of hooked-wire electrodes for electromyography of the intrinsic laryngeal muscles. *J Speech Hear Res.* 1969;12:361–373.

17. Hirano M, Ohala J, Vennard W. The function of laryngeal muscles in regulating fundamental frequency and intensity of phonation. *J Speech Hear Res.* 1969;12:616–628.

18. Hirano M, Vennard W, Ohala J. Regulation of register, pitch and intensity of voice. *Folia Phoniatr.* 1970;22:1–20.

19. Hirose H, Gay T, Strome M. Electrode insertion techniques for laryngeal electromyography. *J Acoust Soc Am.* 1971;50:1449–1450.

20. Hirose H. Clinical observations on 600 cases of recurrent laryngeal nerve palsy. *Annual Bull RILP* (Research Institute of Logopedics and Phoniatrics). University of Tokyo. 1977;11:165–173.

21. Hiroto I, Hirano M, Toyozumi Y, Shin T. A new method of placement of a needle electrode in the intrinsic laryngeal muscles for electromyography insertion through the skin. *Pract Otol (Kyoto).* 1962;55:499–504.

22. Hiroto I, Hirano M, Tomita H. Electromyographic investigation of human vocal cord paralysis. *Ann Otol Rhinol Laryngol.* 1968;77:296–304.

23. Jonsson B, Reichmann S. Displacement and deformation of wire elctrodes in electromyography. *Electromyography.* 1969;9:210–211.

24. Knutsson E, Martensson A, Martensson B. The normal electromyogram in human vocal fold muscles. *Acta Otolaryngol (Stockh).* 1969;68: 526–536.

25. Martensson A, Skoglund CR. Contraction properties of intrinsic laryngeal muscles. *Acta Phys Scand.* 1964;60:318–336.

26. Shipp T, Doherty T, Morrissey P. Predicting vocal frequency from selected physiologic measures. *J Acoust Soc Am.* 1979;66:678–684.

27. Sussman HM, McNeilage PG, Powers RK. Recruitment and discharge patterns of single motor units during speech production. *J Speech Hear Res.* 1977;20:613–630.

28. Yanagihara N, von Leden H. The cricothyroid muscle during phonation—electromyographic, aerodynamic and acoustic studies. *Ann Otol Rhinol Laryngol.* 1968;75:987–1006.

29. Arnold G. Physiology and pathology of the cricothyroid muscle. *Laryngoscope.* 1961;71:687–753.

30. Hirano M. The function of the intrinsic laryngeal muscles in singing. In: Stevens K, Hirano M, eds. *Vocal Fold Physiology.* Tokyo, Japan: University of Tokyo Press; 1981:155–167.

31. Hirano M. Electromyography of laryngeal muscles. In: Hirano M, ed. *Clinical Examination of Voice.* New York, NY: Springer-Verlag; 1981; 11–24.

32. Hirano M. Examination of vocal fold vibration. In: Hirano M, ed. *Clinical Examination of the Voice.* New York, NY: Springer-Verlag; 1981;43–65.

33. Hirose H, Kobayashi T, Okamura M, Kurauchi Y, et al. Recurrent laryngeal nerve palsy. *J Otolaryngol (Japan).* 1967;70:1–17.

34. Khan A, Pearlman RC, Bianchi DA, Hauck KW. Experience with two types of electromyography monitoring electrodes during thyroid surgery. *Am J Otolaryngol.* 1997;18:99–102.

35. Guindi GM, Higenbottam TW, Payne JK. A new method for laryngeal electromyography. *Clin Otolaryngol.* 1981;6:271–278.

36. Fujita M, Ludlow CL, Woodson GE. A new surface electrode for recording from the posterior cricoarytenoid muscle. *Laryngoscope.* 1989; 99:316–320.

37. Andrews S, Warner J, Stewart R. EMG biofeedback in the treatment of hyperfunctional dysphonia. *Br J Disord Commun.* 1986;21:353–369.

38. Hillel AD, Robinson LR, Waugh P. Laryngeal electromyography for the diagnosis and management of swallowing disorders. *Otolaryngol Head Neck Surg.* 1997;116(3):344–348.

39. Brown WF. *The Physiological and Technical Basis of Electromyography.* Stoneham, MA: Butterworth Publishers; 1984.

40. Lovelace RE, Blizter A, Ludlow C. Clinical laryngeal electromyography. In: Blitzer A, Brin MF, Sasaki CT. *Neurologic Disorders of the Larynx.* New York, NY: Thieme; 1992:66–82.

41. Aminoff MJ. Clinical electromyography. In: Aminoff MJ, ed., *Electrodiagnosis in Clinical Neurology.* 4th ed. Philadelphia, Pa: Churchill Livingstone; 1999:223–252.

42. Campbell WW. Needle electrode examination. In: Campbell WW, ed. *Essentials of Neurodiagnostic Medicine.* Baltimore, Md: Williams & Wilkins; 1999:93–116.

43. Basmajian JV, Stecko G. A new bipolar electrode for electromyography. *J Applied Physiol.* 1962;17:849.

44. Blitzer A, Lovelace RE, Brin MF, Fahn S, Fink ME. Electromyographic findings in focal laryngeal dystonia (spasmodic dysphonia). *Ann Otol Rhinol Laryngol.* 1985;94:591–594.

45. Thumfart WF. Electromyography of the larynx and related technics. *Acta Otorhinolaryngol Belg.* 1986;40:358–376.

46. Woo P, Arandia H. Intraoperative laryngeal electromyographic assessment of patients with immobile vocal fold. *Ann Otol Rhinol Laryngol.* 1992;101(10):799–806.

47. Blitzer A, Brin M, Sasaki C. *Neurological Disorders of the Larynx.* New York, NY: Thieme; 1992.

48. Lindestad PA, Persson A. Quantitative analysis of EMG interference pattern in patients with laryngeal paresis. *Acta Oto Laryngologica.* 1994;114(1):91–97.

49. Lindestad PA. *Electromyographic and Laryngoscopic Studies of Normal and Disturbed Voice Function.* Stockholm, Sweden: Departments of Logopedics and Phoniatrics and Clinical Neurophysiology, Huddinge University Hospital; 1994.

50. Titze IR, Luschei ES, Hirano M. The role of the thyroarytenoid muscles in the regulation of fundamental frequency. *J Voice.* 1989;3:213–224.

51. Ludlow C. Neurophysiological control of vocal fold adduction and abduction for phonation onset and offset during speech. In: Gauffin J, Hammarberg B, eds. *Vocal Fold Physiology—Acoustic, Perceptual and Physiological Aspects of Voice Mechanisms.* San Diego, Calif: Singular Publishing Group; 1991:197–205.

52. Willison R. Analysis of electrical activity in healthy and dystrophic muscles in man. *J Neurol Neurosurg Psychiatry.* 1964;27:386–394.

53. Fuglsang-Frederiksen A, Mansson A. Analysis of electrical activity of normal muscle in man at different degrees of voluntary effort. *J. Neurol Neurosurg Psychiatry.* 1975;38:683–694.

54. Philipsson L, Larsson P. The electromyographical signal as a measure of muscular force: a comparison of detection and quantification techniques. *Electromyogr Clin Neurophysiol.* 1988;28:141-150.

55. Stalberg E, Chu J, Bril V, Nandedkar S, Stalberg S, Ericsson M. Automatic analysis of the EMG interference pattern. *Electroencephalogr Clin Neurophysiol.* 1983;56:672-681.

56. Rose A, Willison R. Quantitative electromyography using automatic analysis: studies in healthy subjects and patients with primary muscle disease. *J Neurol Neurosurg Psychiatry.* 1967;30:403-410.

57. Hayward M. Automatic analysis of the electromyogram in healthy subjects of different ages. *J Neurol Sci.* 1977;33:397-413.

58. Fuglsang-Frederiksen A, Lo Monaco M, Dahl K. Turns analysis (peak ratio) in EMG using mean amplitude as a substitute of force measurement. *Electroencephalogr Clin Neurophysiol.* 1985;60:225-227.

59. Fuglsang-Frederiksen A, Scheel U, Buchtal F. Diagnostic yield of the analysis of the pattern of electrical activity of muscle and of individual motor unit potentials in neurogenic involvement. *J Neurol Neurosurg Psychiatry.* 1977;40:544-554.

60. Fuglsang-Frederiksen A. Quantitative electromyography-II. modifications of the turns analysis. *Electromyogr Clin Neurophysiol.* 1987;27: 335-338.

61. Gilchrist JM, Sanjeev D, Nandedkar SD, et al. Automatic analysis of the electromyographic interference pattern using the turns amplitude ratio. *Electroenc Clin Neurophysiol.* 1988;70:534-540.

62. Fuglsang-Frederiksen A, Ronager J. EMG power spectrum, turns-amplitude analysis and motor unit potential duration in neuromuscular disorders. *J Neurol Sci.* 1990;97:81-91.

63. Driscoll BP, Graeco C, Coelho C, et al. Laryngeal function in postpolio patients. *Laryngoscope.* 1995;105(1):35-41.

64. Abaza M, Sataloff RT, Hawkshaw MJ, Mandel S. Laryngeal manifestations of post poliomyelitis syndrome. *J Voice.* 2001;14(3):291-294.

65. Robinson LR, Hille AD, Waugh PF. New laryngeal muscles weakness in postpolio syndrome. *Laryngoscope.* 1988;108(5):732-734.

66. Guindi GM, Bannister R, Gibson WP, Payne JK. Laryngeal electromyography in multiple system atrophy with autonomic failure. *J Neurol Neurosurg Psychiatry.* 1981;44:49-53.

67. Isozaki E, Osanai R, Horiguchi S, Hayashida T, Hirose K, Tanabe H. Laryngeal electromyography with separated surface electrodes in patients with multiple system atrophy presenting with vocal cord paralysis. *J Neurol.* 1994;241:551-556.

68. Dray TG, Robinson LR, Hillel AD. Laryngeal electromyographic findings in Charcot-Marie-Tooth disease type II. *Arch Neurol.* 1999;56: 863–865.

69. Palmer JB, Holloway AM, Tanaka E. Detecting lower motor neuron dysfunction at the pharynx and larynx with electromyography. *Arch Phys Med Rehabil.*1991;72(3):214–218.

70. Quiney RE. Laryngeal electromyography: a useful technique for the investigation of vocal cord palsy. *Clin Otolaryngol.* 1989:14(4) 305–316.

71. Simpson DM, Sternman D, Graves-Wright J, Sanders I. Vocal cord paralysis: clinical and electrophysiologic features. *Muscle Nerve.* 1993; 16(9):925–927.

72. Koufman JA, Postma GN, Cummins MM, Blalock FD. Vocal fold paresis. *Otolaryngol Head Neck Surg.* 2000;122(4)537–541.

73. Parnes SM, Satya-Murti S. Predictive value of laryngeal electromyography in patients with vocal cord paralysis of neurogenic origin. *Laryngoscope.* 1985;95:1323–1326.

74. Tanaka S, Hirano M, Chijiwa K. Some aspects of vocal fold bowing. *Ann Otol Rhinol Laryngol.* 1994;103:357–362.

75. Dursun G. Sataloff RT, Spiegel JR, Mandel S, Heuer RJ, Rosen DC. Superior laryngeal nerve paresis and paralysis. *J Voice.* 1996;10(2):206–211.

76. Dray TG, Robinson LR, Hillel AD. Idiopathic bilateral vocal fold weakness. *Laryngoscope.* 1999;109:995–1002.

77. Gupta SR, Bastian RW. Use of laryngeal electromyography in prediction of recovery after vocal fold paralysis [letter to editor]. *Muscle Nerve.* 1993;16(9):977–978.

78. Min YB, Finnegan EM, Hoffman HT, Luschei ES, McCulloch TM. A preliminary study of the prognostic role of electromyography in laryngeal paralysis. *Otolaryngol Head Neck Surg.* 1994;111(6):770–775.

79. Rodriguez AA, Myers BR, Ford CN. Laryngeal electromyography in the diagnosis of laryngeal nerve injuries. *Arch Phys Med Rehab.* 1990; 71(8)587–590.

80. Hirano M, Nosoe I, Shin T, Maeyama T. Electromyography for laryngeal paralysis. In: Hirano M, Kirchner J, Bless D., eds. *Neurolaryngology: Recent Advances.* Boston, Mass: College-Hill Press; 1987:232–248.

81. Thumfart W. Electromyography of the larynx. In: Samii M, Gannetta PJ, eds. *The Cranial Nerves.* Berlin, Germany: Springer-Verlag; 1981: 597–606.

82. Siribodhi C, Sundmaker W, Adkins JP, Bonner FJ. Electromyographic studies of laryngeal paralysis and regeneration of laryngeal motor nerves in dogs. *Laryngoscope.* 1963;73:148–163.

83. Blitzer A, Jahn AF, Keidar A. Semon's law revisited: an electromyographic analysis of laryngeal synkinesis. *Ann Otol Rhinol Laryngol.* 1996;105:764–769.

84. Gartlan MG, Peterson KL, Luschei ES, Hoffman HT, Smith RJ. Bipolar hooked-wire electromyographic technique in the evaluation of pediatric vocal cord paralysis. *Ann Otol Rhinol Laryngol.* 1993;102(9):695–700.

85. Koch BM, Milmoe G, Grundfast KM. Vocal cord paralysis in children studied by monopolar electromyography. *Ped Neurol.* 1987;3(5):288–293.

86. Berkowitz RG. Laryngeal electromyographic findings in idiopathic congenital bilateral vocal cord paralysis. *Ann Otol Rhinol Laryngol.* 1996;3:207–212.

87. Hoffman HT, Brunberg JA, Winter P, Sullivan MJ, Kileny PR. Arytenoid subluxation: diagnosis and treatment. *Ann Otol Rhinol Laryngol.* 1991;101(1):1–19.

88. Rontal E, Rontal M, Silverman B, Kileny PR. The clinical difference between vocal cord paralysis and vocal cord fixation using electromyography. *Laryngoscope.* 1993;103(2):133–137.

89. Woo P, Arandia H. Intraoperative laryngeal electromyographic assessment of patients with immobile vocal fold. *Ann Otol Rhinol Laryngol.* 1992;101(10):799–806.

90. Sataloff RT, Bough ID, Spiegel JR. Arytenoid dislocation: diagnosis and treatment. *Laryngoscope.* 1994;104(10):1353–1361.

91. Yin SS, Qiu WW, Stucker FJ. Value of electromyography in differential diagnosis of laryngeal joint injuries after intubation. *Ann Otol Rhinol Laryngol.* 1996;105:446–451.

92. Lipton RJ, McCafferty TV, Litchy WJ. Intraoperative electrophysiologic monitoring of laryngeal muscle during thyroid surgery. *Laryngoscope.* 1988;98(12):1292–1296.

93. Khan A, Pearlman RC, Bianchi DA, Hauck KW. Experience with two types of electromyographic monitoring electrodes during surgery. *Am J Otolaryngol.* 1997;18(2):99–122.

94. Benninger MS, Gillen JB, Altman JS, et al. Changing etiology of vocal fold immobility. *Laryngoscope.* 1998;108(9):1346–1350.

95. Koda J, Ludlow CL. An evaluation of laryngeal muscle activation in patients with voice tremor. *Otolaryngol Head Neck Surg.* 1992;107(5):684–696.

96. Smith A, Luschei E, Denny M, Wood J, Hirano M, Badvlak S. Spectral analyses of activity of laryngeal and orofacial muscles in stutterers. *J Neurol Neurosurg Psychiatry.* 1993;56(12):1303–1311.

97. Blitzer A, Lovelace RE, Brin MF, Fahn S, Fink ME. Electromyographic findings in focal laryngeal dystonia (spastic dysphonia). *Ann Otol Rhinol Laryngol.* 1985;94:591-594.

98. Shipp T, Izdebski K, Reed C, Morrissy P. Intrinsic laryngeal muscle activity in a spastic dysphonia patient. *J Speech Hear Dis.* 1985; 50(1):54-59.

99. Blitzer A, Brin M, Fahn S, Lovelace RE. Clinical and laboratory characteristics of focal laryngeal dystonia: study of 110 cases. *Laryngoscope.* 1988;98:636-640.

100. Watson BV, Schaefer SD, Freeman FJ, Dembowski J, Kondraske G, Roark R. Laryngeal electromyographic activity in adductor and abductor spasmodic dysphonia. *J Speech Hear Res.* 1991;34(3):473-482.

101. Rodriquez AA, Ford CN, Bless DM, Harmon RL. Electromyographic assessment of spasmodic dysphonia patients prior to botulinum toxin injection. *Electromyogr Clin Neurophysiol.* 1994;34(7):403-407.

102. Andrews S, Warner J, Steward R. EMG biofeedback and relaxation in the treatment of hyperfunctional dysphonia. *Br J Disord Commun.* 1986;21(3):353-363.

103. Davidson BJ, Ludlow CL. Long-term effects of botulinum toxin injections in spasmodic dysphonia. *Ann Otol Rhinol Laryngol.* 1996; 105(1):33-42.

104. Mao V, Abaza M, Spiegel J, et al. Laryngeal myasthenia gravis: report of 40 cases. *J Voice.* 2001;15(1):122-130.

105. Ertekin C, Avdogdu I, Yuceyar N, et al. Effects of bolus volume on oropharyngeal swallowing: an electrophysiologic study in man. *Am J Gastroenterol.* 1997;92(22):2049-2053.

106. Atkinson SI, Rees J. Botulinum toxin for endopharyngeal dysphagia: case reports of CT-guided injection. *J Otolaryngol.* 1997;26(4): 273-276.

107. Chained CM, Ludlow CL. Single motor unit activity in human intrinsic laryngeal muscles during respiration. *Ann Oto Rhinol and Laryngol.* 1992;101(10):832-840.

108. Brancatisano A, Dodd DS, Engel LA. Posterior cricoarytenoid activity and glottic size during hypernea in humans. *J Appl Physiol.* 1991;71(3):977-982.

109. Kung ST, Insalaco G, Villeponteauz RD. Aryteroideus muscle activity in normal adult humans during wakefulness and sleep. *J Appl Physiol.* 1991;70(4):1655-1664.

110. Eichenwald EC, Howel RO, Kosch PC, Ungarel RA, Lindsey J, Strark R. Developmental changes in sequential activation of laryngeal abductor muscle and diaphragm in infants. *J Appl Physiol.* 1992;73(4): 1425-1431.

111. Insalaco G, Kuna ST, Catania G, et al. Thyroarytenoid muscle activity in sleep apneas. *J Appl Physiol.* 1993;74(2):704–709.

112. Brodiatowski M, Grundfest-Brodiatrowski S, Davies CR, Jacob GB, Tucker HM Nose Y. Electronic pacing of incapacitated head and neck structures. *ASAIO Transactions.* 1991;37(4):553–558.

113. Koufman JA, Postma GN, Whang CH, et al. Diagnostic laryngeal electromyography: the Wake Forest experience 1995–1999. *Otolaryngol Head Neck Surg.* 2001;124(6):603–606.

114. Sataloff RT, Mandel S, Mann EA, Ludlow CL. Practice Parameter: Laryngeal electromyography (an evidence-based review). *J Voice.* 2004; 18(2): 261–274.

CHAPTER 6

Clinical Applications of Laryngeal Electromyography: Case Studies

This chapter illustrates some of the neurolaryngologic problems encountered commonly in clinical practice, as well as the various treatment options and the benefit of laryngeal electromyography in the assessment and treatment processes. These patients were evaluated initially by the authors, laryngologist (RTS and YDH), neurologist (SM and RME) who performed the LEMGs "blinded," that is, without clinical information provided by the laryngologist. We have studied more than 2,000 patients in this fashion and are currently preparing to publish our experience with laryngeal electromyography in a clinical setting. The following cases were selected from this large group of patients to illustrate typical clinical applications of laryngeal EMG.

CASE 1

A 43-year-old white female presented initially to the author (RTS) with complaints of persistent hoarseness, breathiness, and vocal fatigue. She was a high school choral director and choral singer who had a history of two to three episodes of total voice loss per year for the past several years. Her latest episode had occurred two months previously and her voice had not recovered completely. She reported generalized body fatigue, stating that she was "always tired." She also complained of difficulties with the middle range of her singing voice during these episodes. Her past medical history included peptic ulcer disease, mitral valve prolapse, herpes simplex, and herpes zoster. Her past surgical history included exploratory laparotomy for a bleeding ulcer 19 years previously and foot surgery 24 years previously. Her daily medications included an oral contraceptive, H2-blocker, and metoprolol; she was allergic to codeine. She had a 12 pack-year history of smoking, but had quit 16 years ago.

Her head and neck examination was unremarkable. Strobo-videolaryngoscopy using flexible and rigid endoscopes revealed fluctuations in vocal fold mobility. Initially during her examination, the right vocal fold appeared weak and the left appeared normal. However, during the course of the examination the side of weakness appeared to switch. Also noted was a broad-based, fluid-filled mass encompassing the middle third of the right vocal fold. A soft mass was present on the contralateral side, which appeared to be reactive swelling. Mucosal waves were normal, but there was intermittently incomplete glottic closure anterior and posterior to the masses.

General neurologic examination was normal. Laryngeal EMG using monopolar concentric electrodes revealed a 70% reduced recruitment response from both cricothyroid muscles. Recruitment responses from the posterior cricoarytenoid and thyroarytenoid muscles were normal bilaterally. No fibrillations, positive sharp waves, or polyphasic units were detected. Administration of 10 mg of Tensilon (edrophonium) intravenously resulted in a subjective improvement in the patient's voice and electrical improvement on LEMG. Repetitive stimulation of the spinal accessory nerve was abnormal before Tensilon administration, but normal after Tensilon.

The electrical studies were consistent with myasthenia gravis, an autoimmune disorder of the neuromuscular junction. Serum laboratory evaluation revealed a positive FTA-abs but no acetylcholine receptor or skeletal muscle antibodies were detected. Follow-up with MHA-TP was negative. The patient was started on pyridostigmine bromide (Mestinon) 60 mg three times daily and obtained symptomatic relief. Her dose was adjusted to 60 mg three times daily plus 90 mg at bedtime for maximal control of symptoms. When she tried stopping the Mestinon, her dysphonia and vocal fatigue returned; they resolved again when the Mestinon was restarted. She also underwent voice therapy. On follow-up examination 10 months later, improvements in abduction and adduction were seen bilaterally, and the left vocal fold mass had resolved. Fluctuating asymmetries of vocal fold motion were no longer observed.

CASE 2

A 40-year-old marketing executive and avocational musical theater singer had been an active performer since his youth. He had had several years of vocal training, but none in the past 15 to 20 years. Approximately one year prior to evaluation, he noticed hoarseness, decreased range, dryness, breathiness, and a general sense that his voice was "not working right." His past medical history was significant for Lyme disease, which had been diagnosed and treated following a target rash on his chest one year prior to his examination. His dysphonia began at about the same time.

Strobovideolaryngoscopy revealed markedly diminished mobility of the right vocal fold in abduction and adduction, resulting in incomplete glottic closure. Longitudinal tension of both vocal folds appeared to be within normal limits. The patient also had reflux laryngitis. His voice was hoarse, breathy, and intermittently pressed, as is characteristic of compensatory muscular tension dysphonia with supraglottic hyperfunction.

Laryngeal electromyography revealed 80% recruitment response in the distribution of the right superior laryngeal nerve with a few fibrillation potentials and positive sharp waves. The right recurrent nerve showed only 10% recruitment response and had fibrillation potentials, positive sharp waves, and polyphasic units. These findings are consistent with a chronic denervating neuropathy. The left side was normal. The patient was unable to compensate for glottic incompetence through voice and singing therapy alone. This was anticipated on the basis of his LEMG, and attempts at therapy were not prolonged after he had reached a plateau following about five sessions. Autologous fat injection in the right vocal fold resulted in excellent improvement in glottic closure and, subsequently, reduced his muscle tension dysphonia. Approximately 1 year following fat injection, he developed an upper respiratory infection, after which he had slight recurrent and persistent dysphonia. Examination revealed partial fat resorption, which had not been present prior to the upper respiratory infection. A second fat injection was performed, and he has been asymptomatic during the intervening 3 years.

CASE 3

A 25-year-old female chemist, dancer, and recording artist of Polish folk music presented for evaluation of persistent and recurrent voice difficulties over the past several years. She also taught folk music and dance to children three evenings a week, in addition to working full-time as a chemist. Polish was her native language, but she had an excellent mastery of English. She reported having had repeated upper respiratory infections associated with voice loss, and over the past few years, her vocal range had diminished. She also admitted to morning hoarseness, vocal fatigue, occasional throat tickle when she sang, and intermittent hoarseness. She cleared her throat frequently. Her symptoms were more prominent when speaking Polish than they were when speaking English. She had had no formal singing or speaking training. She was in good health otherwise with no history of surgery or illnesses other than mild allergies. She used birth control pills as her only medication. Strobovideolaryngoscopy revealed sluggishness of the left vocal fold, muscle tension dysphonia, soft bilateral vocal fold swellings in the striking zones, and signs of reflux laryngitis. Laryngeal electromyography showed a 70 to 80% recruitment response in the distribution of the left superior laryngeal nerve. Voice therapy was directed at strengthening the weakened neuromuscular complex by elimination of compensatory hyperfunction and by utilizing specific stretching and strengthening exercises directed at the cricothyroid muscle. The patient was also treated for reflux laryngitis and received therapy for her speaking voice and training in singing. Her symptoms resolved entirely, and her voice has remained strong and dependable in the subsequent 2 years. However, clinical examination showed persistent left superior laryngeal nerve paresis for which she had compensated well. Laryngeal EMG was not repeated to confirm this observation, as it would not have altered treatment in this asymptomatic patient.

CASE 4

A 37-year-old professional gospel singer and intensive care unit nurse had studied singing for 7 years prior to her assessment in our office. At age 28, she noticed a change in the pitch of her voice and had transformed from a lyric soprano to a mezzo-soprano. Her voice continued to deepen, was inconsistent, and fatigued easily. She had been diagnosed with asthma several years prior and was treated with corticosteroids and bronchodilator inhalers. However, she had stopped them in favor of a medicinal herb. Three weeks prior to evaluation, she developed an upper respiratory infection and noted gradually increasing hoarseness since that time. At the same time, she had stopped acyclovir (Zovirax), which she had been taking for 3 years for herpes simplex virus (HSV) type I and II. The upper respiratory tract infection had also been associated with exacerbation of her asthma symptoms, and she had resumed using inhalers. The inhalers did not appear to affect her vocal quality or endurance, subjectively. Her medical history also included hypertension and obesity. She weighed approximately 360 lbs (164 kg) and was 5 ft, 6 in (169 cm) tall. She was taking enalapril (Vasotec), progesterone supplements, and the asthma medications noted above. She also used continuous positive airway pressure for sleep apnea and was under treatment for hypoglycemia, hypertension, and a cardiac arrhythmia. Strobovideolaryngoscopy revealed a broad-based, cystic, posthemorrhagic right vocal fold mass and a smaller reactive mass on the left. Initially, there appeared to be left superior laryngeal nerve paresis. However, the symmetry of vocal fold motion appeared to fluctuate throughout the examination. There were also signs of severe reflux laryngitis. Laryngeal electromyography revealed markedly reduced recruitment response with severe fluctuations during the EMG study. There was a 21% decremental response during accessory nerve stimulation. After 10 mg of Tensilon, repetitive stimulation showed only a 2% decrement, and laryngeal EMG response improved markedly. Additionally, the patient reported significant improvement in her voice that lasted for about 5 minutes. She described the changes as "dramatic." She was treated with 300 mg of Mestinon daily, antireflux therapy, and voice therapy. She was referred for pulmonary evaluation, with the goal of eliminating the inhalers and converting her management to oral medications alone. With excellent reflux control, her asthma became asymptomatic, even during singing. Her voice fatigue resolved on Mestinon, her range improved, and she was able to resume singing professionally. In addition, once the chronic fatigue had been improved on Mestinon, she became more successful in her attempts to lose weight.

CASE 5

A 64-year-old woman presented with vocal difficulties that began immediately following a left hemithyroidectomy. Her medical history included nephrectomy for renal cell carcinoma, cholecystectomy, lumbar spinal fusion, basal cell carcinoma of the nose, and removal of benign breast lesions. She had awakened in the recovery room with a hoarse and breathy voice. Other reported symptoms included morning hoarseness, bitter taste, and globus sensation. The operative report described extensive inflammatory reaction and scarring adjacent to the recurrent laryngeal nerve, but noted that the nerve was intact at the end of the procedure. The pathology report described diffuse thyroiditis without malignancy. She had been evaluated by another otolaryngologist who diagnosed left vocal fold paralysis and referred her for voice evaluation and additional therapy six months postoperatively. She had attended only one voice therapy session but practiced her prescribed exercises at home, with no subjective improvement. Strobovideolaryngoscopy revealed left vocal fold immobility, with an absent jostle sign. The left vocal fold was stretched and elevated, and the vocal process was higher than that on the mobile side. There appeared to be muscle contraction during attempts at adduction and abduction, but without arytenoid movement. There were also signs of reflux laryngitis and severe compensatory muscle tension dysphonia. The clinical diagnosis of left posterior arytenoid dislocation was supported by laryngeal electromyography. The study revealed a 70 to 80% recruitment response in the left cricothyroid muscle, in the distribution of the left recurrent laryngeal nerve (the thyroarytenoid and posterior cricoarytenoid muscles were tested), and 70% reduced recruitment in the distribution of the left superior laryngeal nerve. Although these findings are not normal, the degree of paresis they revealed was insufficient to account for the patient's immobile vocal fold and abnormal vocal process position. Laryngeal computed tomography was not diagnostic. On the basis of these findings, she underwent microlaryngoscopy, which confirmed arytenoid subluxation on the left side. Closed reduction was successful at returning her vocal process to the appropriate height, although mobility was not restored. The voice improved markedly, and the problem was reduced to a simple issue of medialization. Autologous fat injection was performed and resulted in excellent restoration of vocal quality and endurance. She also received additional voice therapy and antireflux therapy preoperatively and postoperatively. She has had no recurrence of voice difficulties during 2 years of follow-up.

CASE 6

The patient was a 68-year-old homemaker with a history of Sjögren's syndrome, irritable bowel syndrome, hypertension, hypoglycemia, migraines, mitral valve disease, cardiac arrhythmias, chronic cough, and rhinorrhea. She sang avocationally and had noted the onset of progressive hoarseness and decreased range in her singing voice and a lowering of her habitual speaking pitch over the past 2 years. She had stopped singing in choirs because of her chronic cough, throat clearing, and recent hoarseness, but was anxious to return to singing. Her medications included alendronate sodium (Fosamax, Merck), conjugated estrogens/medroxyprogesterone acetate

(Prempro, Wyeth), enalapril (Vasotec, Merck), aspirin, lactate, and vitamins. Strobovideolaryngoscopy showed right vocal fold paresis, suggestive of superior laryngeal nerve dysfunction. The patient also had compensatory muscle tension dysphonia, as well as findings consistent with reflux. Laryngeal EMG revealed a 50% reduced recruitment response in the distribution of the right superior laryngeal nerve. This degree of impairment is considered a "borderline" finding. Most patients with a 70 to 80% recruitment do well with voice therapy alone, except some professional singers who typically require surgical medialization to return to vocal performance. Most patients with a 30% recruitment response or worse require surgery in addition to therapy to optimize phonation. Patients with 40 to 60% recruitment response are variable in their response to voice therapy alone and at times require surgical medialization to help limit symptoms of vocal fatigue, vocal instability, and/or decreased protection. In this case, the patient experienced satisfactory improvement through voice therapy and specialized singing training, and she was able to return to choral singing after her cough had been cured with antireflux therapy.

CASE 7

A 66-year-old female presented with a 15-month history of hoarseness. She reported having had primary polio at age 12 with mild residual diaphragm and voice weakness. She had no difficulties until 1968, when she developed respiratory distress requiring intubation and tracheotomy following an upper respiratory tract infection. She was extubated after 2 weeks and had no problems until 1995. At that time, she developed hoarseness associated with a cold. She had had dysphagia with the onset of her voice complaints, but the dysphagia had resolved. Her dysphonia had not improved. Otolaryngologic examination was normal with the exception of the larynx. Strobovideolaryngoscopy revealed an immobile left vocal fold, left superior laryngeal nerve paresis, reflux laryngitis, bilateral Reinke's edema, and compensatory muscle tension dysphonia. Laryngeal electromyography revealed left recurrent laryngeal nerve paresis with occasional single, rapid-fire, giant motor unit potentials. The left superior laryngeal nerve showed a 40 to 50% recruitment response, also with giant motor unit potentials. There was also an unexpected finding of a 70% recruitment response in the distribution of the right recurrent laryngeal nerve. Accessory nerve repetitive stimulation studies were normal. The patient has postpolio syndrome. She was treated with voice therapy, which eliminated hyperfunction, decreased fatigue, and improved loudness. Glottic closure was complete without medialization and likely secondary synkinesis. No deterioration was noted over the following 5 years.

SUMMARY

Laryngeal EMG has proven to be extremely useful clinically. We consider it indispensable to accurate diagnosis of laryngeal movement disorders. The information obtained from laryngeal EMG helps not only with establishing a correct diagnosis, but also in planning optimal treatment.

CHAPTER 7

Electrophysiologic Monitoring of Laryngeal Nerves Intraoperatively

Intraoperative laryngeal electrophysiologic monitoring during skull base, neck, and chest surgery can be beneficial. The introduction of endotracheal tubes with surface electrodes to monitor activity within the thyroarytenoid muscles has contributed greatly to ease of intraoperative electrophysiologic monitoring of the recurrent laryngeal nerves. As a result, electrophysiologic intraoperative monitoring has improved our ability to recognize when the recurrent laryngeal nerve is at risk for injury, thus minimizing postoperative morbidity from recurrent laryngeal nerve palsy associated with skull base, neck, and chest surgery.

LARYNGEAL NERVE INJURY

Injury to the laryngeal nerves is one of the most common complications of thyroid surgery. The incidence of recurrent laryngeal nerve palsy following thyroid and parathyroid surgery has been reported to range from 0.3% to 13%.[1-5] Injury to the superior laryngeal nerve is recognized in fewer than 5% of thyroidectomies.[1] The reported incidences of recurrent and superior laryngeal nerve injuries may underestimate the true incidence of injury. In most series reported in the literature, laryngoscopy was not performed routinely preoperatively or postoperatively. Instead, persistent hoarseness, dysphagia, and airway distress were the most common symptoms that prompted an evaluation. However, even in cases of laryngeal nerve injury that are diagnosed eventually, the surgeon was aware that an injury occurred in only one in ten cases.[6,7] In all probability, cases of temporary laryngeal nerve palsy, superior laryngeal nerve injury, and paresis following thyroidectomy were likely underestimated in that series. It is our practice to perform laryngoscopy both preoperatively and postoperatively and laryngeal electromyography preoperatively in all elective thyroid and parathyroid surgeries. In some cases, a pre-existing palsy exists, and it is helpful to identify such abnormalities preoperatively, as these nerves may have been stressed by the thyroid condition, either through stretch, inflammation, or scarring, and are at increased risk for further injury with manipulation of the tissue adjacent to the nerves. We use intraoperative laryngeal nerve monitoring in essentially all cases.

Although superior and recurrent laryngeal nerve injuries occur most commonly following thyroid surgery, they also may occur with any operation that manipulates tissue in the region of the superior laryngeal nerve, recurrent laryngeal nerve, or upper vagus nerve. Such procedures include parathyroid surgery, skull base surgery near the jugular foramen, fusion of the cervical spine via an anterior approach, carotid endarterectomy, coronary artery bypass surgery, aortic artery surgery, Zenker's diverticulectomy, laryngotracheal reconstruction, and other skull base, neck, and chest/upper mediastinal procedures. There is an increased risk of injury in patients with atypical anatomy of the recurrent laryngeal nerves particularly on the right side, in patients with extensive disease processes, in those who have had previous surgery in the current operative field, and in those with a history of irradiation therapy.[5] Particular diligence is necessary in these cases, and intraoperative monitoring of the laryngeal nerves can be a useful adjunct in helping the surgeon protect the laryngeal nerves from injury.

ELECTROPHYSIOLOGIC MONITORING OF THE LARYNGEAL NERVES

Electrophysiologic monitoring of neural activity has significant implications and applications for protecting the laryngeal nerves. Such monitoring has been used with good success for monitoring other cranial nerves, particularly the VIIth cranial nerve, and it appears to be useful for monitoring the recurrent laryngeal nerves. The primary goals of intraoperative nerve monitoring are to facilitate the identification of the laryngeal nerves, to aid dissection of the nerves, to avoid nerve injury, and to provide prognosis for postoperative nerve function.[2,5,8] Electrophysiologic monitoring is not a substitute for good operative techniques nor does it ensure against nerve injury. Instead, electrophysiologic monitoring should be viewed as an aid that helps to alert the surgeon to nerve irritation, which can be from manipulation of surrounding tissues, manipulation or stretch of the nerve, or spontaneous activity related to the depth of the anesthetic state.

Various techniques for monitoring the recurrent laryngeal nerves intraoperatively have been advocated over the past 35 years. These have included the placement of needle or hooked-wire electrodes directly into the vocalis (for RNL monitoring) or cricothyroid (for SLN monitoring) muscles via endoscopic or percutaneous techniques, to the use of double balloon endotracheal tubes to monitor pressure changes in the glottis, to the use of surface electrodes placed within the endotracheal tube or posterior to the cricoid cartilage in the hypopharynx to monitor activity of the vocalis and posterior cricoarytenoid muscles, respectively.[1,5,9-16] An endotracheal tube integrated with surface electrodes such as that manufactured by Xomed (Jacksonville, Fla), is the easiest to place and least likely to dislodge, making this system favored among most surgeons and anesthesiologists. Because this electrode pair is embedded within the outer surface of the endotracheal tube, placement of the electrodes is performed as the patient is intubated, with rotation of the endotracheal tube to ensure contact of the surface electrodes with the vocal folds.

Once the electrodes are positioned, they are connected to the Xomed nerve integrity monitor (NIM-2) connector box. The anesthesiologist is instructed to avoid the use of nondepolarizing neuromuscular blocking agents throughout the period of nerve monitoring, as these will interfere with the ability to monitor the nerves accurately. Short-term paralysis for intubation is not usually problematic. The ground needle electrodes are placed in the patient at a site away from the larynx and the operative field and connected to the NIM-2 connector box. Impedance values are then checked to ensure proper electrode positioning. Individual impedance values should all be less than 5 kohm with an imbalance of less than 1 kohm. Once optional position of the electrodes has been obtained, the endotracheal tube should be secured to prevent change in electrode position with patient movement. If a stimulating electrode is to be used to confirm identification of the laryngeal nerve, then the constant current stimulation parameters should be set at 4 stimulations per second, stimulus duration of 100 microseconds, and an amplitude of 1 milliamp (MA).[2] Although there have been reports of no signs of injury to the recurrent laryngeal nerve with stimulation intraoperatively at 1 MA, in general, stimulation of the nerve should be avoided unless absolutely necessary, as it has been thought to contribute to temporary paresis.[2]

Because muscle relaxants are not used during electrophysiologic monitoring of the laryngeal nerves, there may be nerve activity observed due to respiratory variation when the patient is in a light plane of anesthesia. This is typically viewed on the oscilloscope as a sawtoothed or jagged increase in baseline activity with waveform amplitudes of 30 to 70 microvolts.[2] This respiratory variation is usually the first sign that the anesthetic state is lightening and is usually soon followed by generalized, involuntary muscle activity and patient movement. When respiratory variation is seen on the oscilloscope, a deeper plane of anesthetic is usually indicated. When the anesthetic state is appropriate, there is minimal baseline activity, with waveform amplitudes of 10 to 20 microvolts. If, during the course of the surgical procedure, the nerve is manipulated directly, a single, polyphasic burst of activity will occur that usually lasts less than 1 second.[8] If the auditory feedback on the NIM-2 is on (which it should always be), this burst will be heard as a single "pop." If the nerve is stretched secondary to manipulation of the surrounding tissues, a train response is seen and heard on the oscilloscope. This train response is characterized by several successive bursts of polyphasic activity with amplitudes greater than 100 microvolts and is heard as a continuous or rapidly successive "popping" sound. Both the train and burst responses cease with cessation of the offending surgical manipulation and activity. A train response that persists despite cessation of manipulation may imply neural injury.[8] A transected nerve may elicit a burst or train response during manipulation (prior to transection), but usually will cease all electrical activity once cut. Stimulation of the nerve with the stimulating probe set at 1 milliamp typically results in a biphasic summation potential that usually has an amplitude of 500 to 800 millivolts.[2]

LIMITATIONS

One of the most important aspects of laryngeal nerve monitoring is that the surgeon must be keenly aware of the notion that the only accurate way to prevent nerve injury is to visualize the nerve directly. Electrophysiologic monitoring is not foolproof, and if used incorrectly it can contribute inadvertently to nerve injury. Before transecting any tissue that is at all questionable, the nerve must be identified clearly. The inability to stimulate tissue with the stimulating probe does not ensure that that tissue is not neural. If no response is obtained, the larynx should be palpated for signs of muscle activity with stimulation, the probe should be checked for malfunction or replaced by a disposable stimulator, position of the endotracheal tube electrodes should be verified, impedances should be checked, the batteries and power supply on the NIM-2 should be evaluated, and the anesthesiologist or nurse anesthetist should be questioned regarding the use of muscle relaxants, particularly if there has been a change of shift during the procedure. Under no circumstances should questionable tissue be cut until after the nerve has been positively identified.

SUMMARY

Electrophysiologic monitoring of the laryngeal nerves can be a useful adjunct in helping the surgeon protect the laryngeal nerves. However, it is not a substitute for good surgical technique and cannot be depended on to prevent laryngeal nerve injury—it does not. Nevertheless, it undoubtedly assists in nerve identification and preservation in many patients, and its use is recommended.

REFERENCES

1. Lipton RJ, McCafferey TV, Litchy WJ. Intraoperative electrophysiologic monitoring of laryngeal muscle during thyroid surgery. *Laryngoscope.* 1988;98:1292-1296.
2. Randolph GW. Surgical anatomy of the recurrent laryngeal nerve. In: Randolph GW, ed. *Surgery of the Thyroid and Parathyroid Glands.* Philadelphia, Pa: Saunders; 2003:300-342.
3. Lo CY, Kwoh KF, Yuen PW: A prospective evaluation of recurrent laryngeal nerve paralysis during thyroidectomy. *Arch Surg.* 2000; 135(2):204-207.
4. Wagner HE, Seiler C. Recurrent laryngeal nerve paralysis after thyroid gland surgery. *Br J Surg.* 1984;81(2):226-228.
5. Eisle DW. Intraoperative electrophysiologic monitoring of the recurrent laryngeal nerve. *Laryngoscope.* 1996;106:443-449.
6. Patlow C, Norton J. Brennan. Vocal cord paralysis and reoperative parathyroidectomy. *Ann Surg.* 1986;203(3):282-285.
7. Holt GR, McMurray GR, Joseph DL. Recurrent laryngeal nerve injury following thyroid operations *Surg Gynecol Obstet.* 1977;144(4): 567-570.
8. Highlander RL, McDaniel SL. Intraoperative monitoring of lower cranial nerves in surgery of the skull base. *Op Tech Otolaryngol Head Neck Surg.* 1996;7:192-199.
9. Flisberg K, Cindholm T. Electrical stimulation of the human recurrent laryngeal nerve during thyroid operation. *Acta Otolaryngol.* 1970; 263:63-67.
10. Rea JL, Davis WE, Templer JW. Recurrent nerve location system. *Ann Otol Rhinol Laryngol.* 1979;88:92-94.
11. Davis WE, Rea JE, Templer JW. Recurrent laryngeal nerve localization using a microlaryngeal electrode. *Otolaryng Head Neck Surg.* 1979; 87:330-333.

12. Rice DH, Cone-Wesson B. Intraoperative recurrent laryngeal nerve monitoring. *Otolaryngol Head Neck Surg.* 1991;105:372–375.

13. Beck DL, Maves MD. Recurrent laryngeal nerve monitoring during thyroid surgery. In: Kartush JM, Bouchard KR, eds. *Neuromonitoring in Otology and Head and Neck Surgery.* New York, NY: Raven Press; 1992:151–155.

14. Maloney RW, Morcek BW, Steehler KW, et al. A new method for intraoperative recurrent laryngeal nerve monitoring. *Ear Nose Throat J.* 1994:73:30–33.

15. Goldstone AC, Schettino RL. The electrode endotracheal tube: a state of the art method for monitoring recurrent laryngeal nerve vocal cord muscle integrity in the intubated patient. *Otolaryngol Head Neck Surg.* 1990;103:249–251.

16. Rea JL. Postcricoid surface laryngeal electrode. *Ear Nose Throat J.* 1992;71:267–269.

APPENDIX I

Laryngeal Electromyography: Summary Outline of Selected and Important Facts

1. Definition and Overview
   A. Laryngeal electromyography (EMG) is a test that evaluates the integrity of the motor system by recording action potentials generated in muscle fibers.
   B. EMG is particularly useful for evaluating disorders affecting the lower motor neurons, peripheral nerves, neuromuscular junction, and muscles.
   C. EMG should be considered an extension of the physical examination, not an isolated laboratory procedure.

D. EMG abnormalities should be interpreted within the context of the clinical impression.

E. A motor unit consists of a lower motor neuron, its axon, and the muscle fibers innervated. EMG measures extracellularly the spatial and temporal summation of all muscle action potentials belonging to a motor unit. This is known as the motor unit potential.

2. Indications for Laryngeal Electromyography

A. Differentiation of vocal fold paralysis from mechanical (cricoarytenoid joint) fixation. If the vocal fold does not move, but laryngeal EMG is normal, it is mechanically fixed, not paralyzed.

B. Evaluation of suspected hysterical dysphonia or malingering. In such cases, abductors and adductors fire simultaneously. This finding can also be seen in some cases of synkinesis, but such neuropathic cases are usually unilateral and associated with muscle weakness. Hysteria/malingering and synkinesis are generally easy to distinguish from one another.

C. Any suspected laryngeal movement disorder
   i. Recurrent laryngeal nerve paresis or paralysis
   ii. Superior laryngeal nerve paresis or paralysis
   iii. Motor neuron disorders
   iv. Laryngeal dystonia
   v. Laryngeal tremor

D. Suspected disorders of neuromuscular transmission

E. Suspected myopathies

F. Laryngeal dystonia (phonatory or respiratory)

G. Aspiration

H. Assessment of neuromuscular function following laryngeal trauma

I. Needle guidance for botulinum toxin injection

3. Techniques

A. Electrodes
   i. Monopolar needle electrodes are sharp needles, insulated except near their tips. A reference electrode is placed at a remote location and may be a surface electrode.
   ii. Concentric electrodes consist of a needle that serves as a reference electrode, and a central, insulated core. The area of sampling is controlled by the angle of the

bevel of the needle. A needle electrode records action potentials from about 2 to 20 muscle fibers within a 1-mm radius from the electrode tip.

   iii. Hooked-wire electrodes are fine wires that are insulated completely except at the tip, which is hooked. They are inserted inside a needle. When the needle is withdrawn, the hooks on the end of the wires act as barbs, stabilizing electrode position within the muscle. They cannot be repositioned once they have been placed, but they are easily removed. The wires form a bipolar electrode. They are well tolerated and can be left in position for long periods of time.

   iv. Surface electrodes are noninvasive, large monopolar electrodes that are attached to the surface of the skin. They are not suitable for diagnostic recording from small muscles such as those found in the larynx.

   v. For laryngeal electromyography, a needle is inserted through the skin, after the skin has been cleaned with alcohol. Electrodes may be placed into any of the laryngeal muscles. Electrodes can also be placed transorally (through the mouth).

B. Instrumentation

   i. Differential amplifier, with a typical common mode rejection ratio of 100,000:1 and a high-input impedance of at least 100,000 kohms.

   ii. Frequency band is typically set at 10 Hz to 10,000 kHz.

   iii. Machine well-grounded to reduce the risk of electrical injury and 60 Hz interference.

   iv. EMG signal is displayed on a cathode ray oscilloscope, and broadcast audibly through a loudspeaker. The signal can be stored permanently on magnetic tape, computer disk, or paper.

C. Interpretation

   i. Qualitative analysis is used most commonly.

   ii. Quantitative assessment is possible.

4. Needle Position

A. Thyroarytenoid muscle: needles placed through the cricothyroid membrane, about 0.5 cm from the midline, angled superiorly 30 to 45 degrees, and inserted approximately 1 cm.

    B. Lateral cricoarytenoid muscle: insertion similar to thyroary-tenoid muscle, but angled more posterolaterally and slightly lower.

    C. Posterior cricoarytenoid muscle: reached either by placing the needle through the airway and out the back of the cricoid cartilage, or behind the thyroid lamina, after rotating the larynx. The posterior cricoarytenoid muscle is located relatively low (inferiorly) in the larynx.

    D. Cricothyroid muscle: external to the cartilage, deep to the skin, placed laterally between the cricoid and inferior portion of the thyroid cartilage.

5. The EMG Examination

    A. Insertional activity: Insertion of the needle causes bursts of electrical activity. They should not last more than several hundred milliseconds.

    B. Spontaneous activity: At rest, no electrical activity should be recorded, except when the electrode is close to the neuromuscular junction. In that case, end plate spikes and noise may be recorded.

    C. Minimal voluntary contraction: With minimal voluntary contraction, 1 or 2 motor unit potentials can be recorded, with a firing rate of 2 to 5 per second. The average duration of motor unit potentials from the laryngeal muscles is 5 to 6 msecs, with an amplitude of 200 to 500 microvolts.

    D. Maximum voluntary contraction: As the intensity of contraction increases, the firing rate of the motor unit potential increases, and new and larger motor units are recruited until the oscilloscope screen is full, and single motor unit potentials cannot be distinguished one from another. This is called a *full interference pattern*.

6. Common Abnormal Laryngeal EMG Findings

    A. Increased insertional activity: insertional bursts of electrical activity lasting more than several hundred milliseconds. This indicates muscle membrane instability, and is associated with myopathic and neurogenic processes. Insertional activity can also be reduced, suggesting loss of muscle fiber and replacement of it by fibrotic tissue or lipoid degeneration. This is typically associated with end-stage myopathic and some neuropathic processes, but it also may be seen following trauma and hemorrhage into a muscle, followed by fibrosis.

B. Abnormal Spontaneous Activity

    i. *Fibrillation potentials* are spontaneous, single-fiber muscle action potentials with typical amplitudes of several hundred microvolts and durations of less than 2 msecs. They fire regularly at 1 to 50 Hz and are typically biphasic or triphasic with an initial positive deflection. They are seen commonly with denervation, and occasionally in myopathic processes.

        Positive sharp waves are single-fiber contractions of an injured muscle fiber. There is a large positive deflection of several hundred microvolts lasting less than 2 msecs, followed by a negative deflection of 10 to 30 msecs, and regular firing at 1 to 50 Hz. Fibrillation potentials and positive sharp waves usually occur together, and they are seen about 2 to 3 weeks after denervation has occurred. After nerve injury, they indicate denervation and axonal loss. Fibrillation potentials and positive sharp waves produce a very characteristic noise in the loudspeaker.

    ii. *Complex repetitive discharges* occur when a group of muscle fibers discharge repetitively, nearly synchronously, through ephaptic activation. Typically, they have an abrupt onset and cessation, and bizarre configuration. The discharge rate ranges between 5 and 100 Hz, and the amplitude ranges from 100 to 1 mvolt. Complex repetitive discharges are associated with both neuropathic and myopathic processes, but they typically indicate chronicity.

    iii. *Myotonic potentials* are repetitive discharges at rates of 20 and 150 Hz and amplitudes of 20 mvolts to 1 mvolt. They are associated with fibrillation potentials or positive sharp waves. The amplitude and frequency of the potentials wax and wane, causing a characteristic "dive bomber" sound in the EMG loudspeaker. They occur spontaneously, with needle insertion, with percussion of the muscle, or with voluntary contractions. They indicate muscle membrane instability and are seen most commonly in disorders of clinical myotonia, such as myotonic dystrophy. Rarely, they can be seen in chronic neurogenic and myopathic processes without myotonia.

C. Abnormalities Seen During Minimal Voluntary Contraction (Used to Evaluate Morphology of Motor Unit Potentials)

　i. In neuropathic processes, the motor unit potential has a prolonged duration and increased number (more than 4) of phases. During early reinnervation, the amplitude is decreased. When reinnervation is completed, the amplitude is increased.

　ii. In myopathic processes, the duration of the motor unit is potentially short, with an increased number of phases and decreased amplitude.

D. Abnormalities with Maximum Muscle Contraction (Used to Evaluate Interference Pattern and Recruitment)

　i. In neuropathic processes, there is decreased recruitment, with fewer motor units firing at high frequency, and decreased interference pattern.

　ii. In myopathic processes, there is rapid and early recruitment with a low voltage, and a full interference pattern in the context of a weak muscle contraction.

E. Repetitive Stimulation

　i. Repetitive stimulation studies involve stimulating muscles with electrical shocks, and recording neuromuscular response by EMG. Under ordinary circumstances, neuromuscular contraction remains strong. If the electrical stimulation causes progressively decreasing response (reduced recruitment response), abnormalities such as neuromuscular junction disorders (myasthenia gravis) should be considered.

F. Tensilon Test

　i. Tensilon may be given intravenously in association with laryngeal electromyography. If laryngeal EMG abnormalities have been identified, especially decreasing or fluctuating recruitment response, Tensilon test may be considered. If infusion of Tensilon results in marked improvement in laryngeal EMG findings, or return to normalcy, neuromuscular junction disorder (myasthenia gravis) should be suspected.

7. Laryngeal EMG Abnormalities in Specific Disease Categories
   A. Lower Motor Neuron Disease
      i. Increased insertional activities.
      ii. Positive waves and fibrillation potentials.
      iii. Complex repetitive discharges and rarely myotonic discharges.
      iv. Prolonged motor unit potential with an increased number of phases. The amplitude can be either increased or decreased.
      v. Incomplete interference pattern with decreased recruitment and rapid firing of the remaining motor units.
      vi. Laryngeal EMG can be useful in the evaluation of hoarseness and dysphagia in patients with lower motor neuron problems such as amyotrophic lateral sclerosis, polio, and postpolio syndrome.
      vii. Extremely valuable in the evaluation of vocal fold palsy to determine degree of denervation, potential for improvement through voice therapy, and potential for and rate of neuromuscular recovery.
      viii. Laryngeal EMG can also be used to prevent lower motor neuron injury by intraoperative monitoring, during thyroid surgery, for example.
   B. Basal Ganglia Disorders
      i. Insertional activity is normal.
      ii. There is no abnormal spontaneous activity. There may be excessive motor unit potential at rest, indicating incomplete muscle relaxation.
      iii. Poor coordination between agonist and antagonist muscles, or inappropriate activation.
      iv. Rhythmic and periodic discharges of motor unit potentials in patients with voice tremor.
      v. In laryngeal dystonia, there are intermittent, sudden increases in muscle activity coinciding with momentary voice arrest.
   C. Muscle Disorders
      i. Insertional activity can be increased or decreased.

      ii. Positive sharp waves and fibrillation potentials are present in some cases, such as myositis and other muscular dystrophies.

     iii. Complex repetitive discharges and myotonic potentials can occur.

     iv. The motor unit potential is short, with an increased number of phases and decreased amplitude.

      v. Recruitment is rapid and early, with a full interference pattern that is of low amplitude.

  D. Neuromuscular Junction Disorders

       i. Insertional activity is normal.

      ii. No spontaneous activity.

     iii. With minimal contraction, motor unit potential exhibits variation in amplitude and duration.

     iv. Recruitment and interference pattern is normal.

      v. Repetitive stimulation studies are abnormal.

  E. Upper Motor Neuron Disorders

       i. Insertional activity is normal.

      ii. No spontaneous activity.

     iii. No polyphasic motor units. Amplitude and duration of motor unit potential are normal.

     iv. There is decreased recruitment and interference pattern.

      v. Firing rate of the motor unit is slow.

8. Highlights

  A. Laryngeal EMG may provide valuable diagnostic information on any patient with a suspected abnormality of vocal fold motion.

  B. Laryngeal EMG may provide prognostic information in patients with vocal fold paralysis.

  C. Laryngeal EMG may help guide voice therapy.

  D. Laryngeal EMG may help determine the nature and timing of surgery in patients with abnormalities of vocal fold motion, or of glottic competence.

  E. Laryngeal EMG may help guide the placement of botulinum toxin, when this agent is used to treat a laryngeal disorder.

APPENDIX II

Practice Parameter: Laryngeal Electromyography (An Evidence-Based Review)

Robert T. Sataloff, Steven Mandel, Eric A. Mann, and Christy L. Ludlow

Philadelphia, Pennsylvania and Bethesda, Maryland

Summary: This paper reports on an evidence-based review of laryngeal electromyography (EMG) as a technique for use in the diagnosis, prognosis, and treatment of laryngeal movement disorders,

Accepted for publication December 23, 2002.

Address correspondence and reprint requests to Robert T. Sataloff, 1721 Pine Street, Philadelphia, PA 19103. E-mail: aiver@uscom.com

Journal of Voice, Vol. 18, No. 2, pp. 261–274

0892-1997/$30.00

© 2004 The Voice Foundation

doi:10.1016/S0892-1997(03)00008-0

including the laryngeal dystonias, vocal fold paralysis, and other neurolaryngological disorders. The authors performed a systematic review of the medical literature from 1944 through 2001 on the clinical application of EMG to laryngeal disorders. Thirty-three of the 584 articles met the predefined inclusion criteria. The evidence demonstrated that in a double-blind treatment trial of botulinum toxin versus saline, laryngeal EMG used to guide injections into the thyroarytenoid muscle in persons with adductor spasmodic dysphonia was beneficial. A crossover comparison between laryngeal EMG-guided injection and endoscopic injection of botulinum toxin into the posterior cricoarytenoid muscle in abductor spasmodic dysphonia found no significant difference between the two techniques and no significant treatment benefit. Based on the evidence, laryngeal EMG is possibly useful for the injection of botulinum toxin into the thyroarytenoid muscle in the treatment of adductor spasmodic dysphonia. There were no evidence-based data sufficient to support or refute the value of laryngeal EMG for the other uses investigated, although there is extensive anecdotal literature suggesting that it is useful for each of them. There is an urgent need for evidence-based research addressing other applications in the use of laryngeal EMG for other applications.

Key Words: Botulinum toxin—Electromyography—Laryngeal dystonias—Laryngeal movement disorders.

INTRODUCTION

Mission statement

Although laryngeal electromyography (EMG) is used today by practitioners, a comprehensive review of its value in the diagnosis, prognosis, and treatment of laryngeal movement disorders has not been undertaken previously. For this reason, the American Association of Electrodiagnostic Medicine (AAEM) established the Laryngeal EMG Task Force to develop a practice parameter to guide clinical utilization of laryngeal EMG.

Background and justification

Development of laryngeal electromyography

Laryngeal EMG was introduced in 1944 by Weddel et al[1] and advanced substantially in the 1950s by Faaborg-Andersen, Buchtal, and others.[2-4] Additional research by various investigators in the 1960s and 1970s began to clarify the potential importance of EMG in laryngology.[5-29]

Many studies were investigations of the role of the laryngeal muscles in speech and voice production[9,16] or were aimed at increased understanding of laryngeal biomechanics.[13-19] Most of these studies used bipolar hooked wire electrodes and did not address a clinical role for the technique. In the later 1980s and the 1990s, laryngeal EMG was added to the laryngologic assessment and treatment of voice disorders.[30-36] The laryngeal EMG procedure is usually performed by a neurologist, physiatrist, or laryngologist skilled in electrodiagnostic medicine. Laryngeal EMG techniques use primarily needle recordings of voluntary activity.

Current uses of laryngeal electromyography and clinical question statements

Laryngeal EMG is currently being used with greater frequency for the diagnosis, prognosis, and treatment of voice disorders. Unfortunately, relatively few professionals trained in EMG have practical experience in laryngeal EMG or a comprehensive understanding of the anatomy and physiology of laryngeal disorders. The AAEM's Laryngeal EMG Task Force identified seven clinical questions that encompass the current common applications of laryngeal EMG as follows:

> Does laryngeal EMG provide accurate diagnostic information for differentiating vocal fold paresis and paralysis from mechanical fixation of the cricoarytenoid joint?

> Does laryngeal EMG provide accurate prognostic information regarding the likelihood of recovery from vocal fold paresis and paralysis?

Is laryngeal EMG accurate in the diagnosis of diseases affecting the neuromuscular junction?

Can laryngeal EMG differentiate malingering or psychogenic dysphonia from normalcy and neurological dysfunction affecting the laryngeal muscles?

Can laryngeal EMG aid in the identification of muscle activation abnormalities in laryngeal dystonias?

Does laryngeal EMG provide accurate diagnostic information of systemic neuropathic and myopathic disorders involving the larynx?

Is laryngeal EMG a beneficial technique for guiding the treatment of laryngeal dystonias?

PROCESS

Panel selection

A panel of experts was selected to serve on the task force and to undertake an evidence-based review of the literature to answer each of the seven clinical questions defined above.

Literature review process

Search terms

The task force conducted a review of the scientific literature supporting the utilization of laryngeal EMG for the diagnosis, prognosis, and treatment of voice disorders. The National Library of Medicine's MEDLINE database was searched from 1966 through January 2001. As recommended in Appendix 4 of the American Academy of Neurology—Therapeutics and Technology Assessment (AANTTA) Process Document,[37] a MEDLINE search was conducted using the terms "laryngeal" and "electromyography" in combinations as follows: "all [larynx or laryngeal] and all [electromyography or EMG]." This initial search was augmented with the search term "botulinum toxin."

Databases

The articles retrieved by the search were sorted according to the proposed uses and questions. Further subsearches for each topic then were used to identify individual articles of interest for classification (class I, II, III, and IV) using the terms "diagnosis" or "sensitivity" or "specificity" or "prognosis."

Inclusion/exclusion criteria and process of selection of articles

The 1999 practice parameter criteria developed by the AAN were followed to classify all articles identified in this evidence-based review.[37] The Criteria of Classification of Article Strength are provided in Table 1. In most cases, the reference standard for diagnosis of laryngeal disorders is laryngeal videostroboscopy with fiberoptic nasolaryngoscopy.

Number of abstract and articles found/excluded

Initially 584 studies were retrieved using the search terms. However, very few were formal studies aimed at establishing the potential use of laryngeal EMG as a diagnostic, therapeutic, or prognostic procedure. To date, 33 articles qualified for inclusion in the Evidence Tables using the criteria in Table 1 for diagnostic, prognostic, and therapeutic studies. None of the articles was class I or class II with regard to laryngeal EMG. Regarding the use of laryngeal EMG for the treatment of laryngeal dystonias, two were class III. All other articles were class IV which were selected for inclusion because they (1) provided sufficient information to allow the reader to understand the methodology clearly enough to repeat the study, (2) used standard clinical and electromyographic techniques, (3) provided information on methods for clinical diagnosis, and (4) either reported a substantial series of 20 or more patients[3,6,22,38,39,40–47] or reported a smaller number of patients illustrating the use of laryngeal EMG for evaluation of specific clinical problems (all other studies). The reference standard is clinical diagnosis, including laryngoscopy. The task force member used the definitions for elements of evidence and classifications of evidence as defined in the AAN-TTA Process Document.[37]

TABLE 1. *Criteria for Classification*

Type	Class of Study	Blinded Evaluation	Cohort Size	Design	Comparison Groups
Diagnostic	I	yes	Broad	prospective	control
Diagnostic	II	yes	Narrow	prospective	control
Diagnostic	II	yes	broad	retrospective	control
Diagnostic	III	yes	narrow	retrospective	control
Diagnostic	IV	no	narrow	retrospective	no

Type	Class of Study	Blinded Evaluation	Cohort Size	Design	Subjects
Prognostic	I	yes	broad	prospective	spectrum at risk
Prognostic	II	yes	narrow	prospective	narrow spectrum at risk
Prognostic	II	yes	broad	retrospective	spectrum at risk
Prognostic	III	yes	narrow	retrospective	narrow spectrum
Prognostic	IV	no	narrow	retrospective	spectrum at risk

Type	Class	Blinded	Groups	Design	Groups Equivalent
Therapeutic	I	yes	Experimental and control	prospective	At baseline
Therapeutic	II	yes	Experimental and control	prospective	matched
Therapeutic	II	yes	Experimental and control	prospective	Experimental and control
Therapeutic	III	no	Pre-post measures	Prospective	Patients are own controls
Therapeutic	IV	no	no	retrospective	no

Development of evidence tables

The evidence results were classified based on the experimental design for each study and compiled in Evidence Tables 2–8 for each of the seven proposed clinical applications for laryngeal EMG. These tables were then used as the basis for establishing recommendations for the various applications.

Internal and external review of the document

Based on the criteria for establishing recommendations used by the AAN-TTA, the following were used in developing a Rating of Recommendation:

> *Recommendation A:* Class I studies are required for establishing a technology as useful or predictive for a given condition in the specified population and require at least one convincing class I study or at least two consistent convincing class II studies.

of Article Strength

Dx or Outcome Mzr	Systematic Application	Measure(s) Used	Sensitivity	Specificity
Reference Standard	yes	Systematic tests	yes	yes
Reference Standard	yes	Systematic tests	yes	yes
Reference Standard	yes	Systematic tests	yes	yes
established	yes	Systematic tests	no	no
no	no	Expert opinion	no	no

Case Definition	Determine	Outcome Measure(s) Used	Sensitivity	Specificity
Reference Standard	Predictive ability	Administered in a blinded fashion	yes	yes
Reference Standard	Predictive ability	Administered in a blinded fashion	yes	yes
Reference Standard	Predictive ability	Administered in a blinded fashion	yes	yes
Reference Standard	Predictive ability	Administered in a blinded fashion	no	no
Reference Standard	Predictive ability	Administered unblinded	no	no

Group Assignment	Exclusion/Inclusion Criteria	Outcome Measure(s) Used	Drop outs Accounted	Cross-overs
randomized	yes	blinded	yes	yes
no	yes	blinded	yes	yes
randomized	yes	blinded	no	no
Not random	yes	Independent from treatment	no	no
no	no	Expert opinion	no	no

Recommendation B: Class II studies are required for classifying a technology as probably useful or predictive for a given condition in the specified population and require at least one convincing class II study or at least three consistent class III studies.

Recommendation C: Class III studies are required for determining that a technology is possibly useful or predictive for a given condition in the specified population and require at least two convincing and consistent class III studies.

Recommendation U: The unknown recommendation is to be used when data are inadequate and the technology is unproven.

ANALYSIS OF THE EVIDENCE

Two studies provide class III evidence that laryngeal EMG may be useful in the treatment of abductor or adductor spasmodic dysphonia.[48,49] Bielamowicz et al[48] conducted a randomized cross-over comparison of the use of laryngeal EMG with the use of endoscopic-

TABLE 2. *Diagnosis of Vocal Fold Paresis and*

Author Year	Class of Study	Blinded Evaluation	Cohort Size	Comparison Groups	Dx Reference Standard or Outcome Mzr
Satoh, 1978 (51)	IV	no	6 selected patients with vocal fold paralysis where EMG was helpful	5 normal controls, 6 patients with paralysis	none
Faaborg-Andersen, 1957 (3)	IV	no	23 patients with vocal fold paralysis	32 normal controls; Compared paretic and normal side	none
Haglund, 1972 (52)	IV	no	10 patients with vocal fold paralysis	Normal control data referenced from prior study	none
Dedo, 1970 (6)	IV	no	49 patients with vocal fold paralysis	compared normal and paretic side; normal control subjects	none
Rontal, 1993 (53)	IV	no	2 patients with immobile vocal folds	Case reports	none
Miller 1984 (54)	IV	no	3 patients with immobile vocal folds	Case reports	none
Lindestad, 1994 (55)	IV	no	10 patients with vocal fold paralysis	6 normal subjects	none
Yin, 2000 (38)	IV	no	34 patients with vocal fold immobility	11 normal control subjects	none
Dray, 1999 (56)	IV	no	4 patients with bilateral vocal fold paresis	no	none
Yin, 1997 (57)	IV	no	6 patients with laryngeal paralysis or C-A joint pathology	no	none
Hiroto, 1968 (22)	IV	no	21 patients with unilateral vocal fold paralysis	no	none
Blair, 1977 (58)	IV	no	19 patients with recurrent and/or SLN palsy; 6 of these were bilateral	no	none
Koufman, J.A., 2001 (40)	IV	no	415 patients undergoing LEMG for suspected neuromuscular disorder	no	none
Haglund, 1973 (59)	IV	no	9 patients with idiopathic vocal fold paralysis	no	none
Hirano, 1987 (41)	IV	no	110 cases of unilateral vocal fold paralysis	no	none

guided injection for the treatment of abductor spasmodic dysphonia by botulinum toxin injections into the posterior cricoarytenoid muscle. Blinded measures demonstrated no significant reduction in breathy breaks with either technique and no differences between the techniques in abductor spasmodic dysphonia. A study by Ludlow et al[49] used laryngeal EMG to administer botulinum toxin

Paralysis versus Mechanical Fixation or Normal

Systematic Application	Measure(s) Used	Sensitivity	Specificity
Stimulation of the vagus, superior laryngeal nerve and recurrent nerves	Evoked muscle response	N/A	N/A
Concentric needle electrode EMG	MUP duration and amplitude	N/A	N/A
Concentric needle EMG	MUP duration and amplitude, interference pattern	All EMG recordings showed evidence of denervation	N/A
Bipolar concentric	Absence of MUP or fibrillations	All EMG recordings showed evidence of denervation	N/A
Bipolar concentric	No measures	NA	NA
Concentric needle	Presence of MUP and fibrillation potentials	N/A	N/A
Compared conventional and quantitative EMG	Clinical judgement of interference pattern in conventional Turns/s at different amplitudes in quantitative	Conventional 66% Quantitative 33%	Conventional 25% Quantitative 50%
Concentric needle	not specified, no quantitative data	N/A	N/A
monopolar electrode	waveform morphology, voluntary MUP	N/A	N/A
monopolar	not specified, no quantitative data	N/A	N/A
not stated	waveform morphology, recruitment patterns, no quantitative data	N/A	N/A
concentric	waveform morphology, interference pattern, synkinesis	90% demonstrated some abnormality on LEMG	N/A
bipolar needle	waveform morphology, recruitment	11/19 (58%)showed evidence of denervation	N/A
monopolar	recruitment, waveform morphology, spontaneous activity, synkinesis	differentiated fixation from paralysis in 49 patients (12%)	not assessed
not specified	MUP amplitude, duration and interference pattern	N/A	N/A
bipolar needle	waveform morphology, interference pattern	35% showed silence or fibrillations	12% of studies showed no abnormality

injections into the thyroarytenoid muscle in adductor spasmodic dysphonia with a blinded comparison of baseline and posttreatment speech measures. This study demonstrated a significant improvement in speech after treatment. Truong et al[50] performed a double-blinded, randomized, placebo-controlled study of botulinum toxin injection treatment of patients with adductor spasmodic dysphonia.

TABLE 3. *Prognosis for Vocal Fold Paresis*

Author Year	Class of Study	Blinded Evaluation	Cohort Size	Comparison Groups	Outcome Measure
Sittel, 2001 (42)	IV	Outcome measure was not blinded to EMG findings	98 patients with vocal fold paralysis	Prognostic study	Free vocal fold mobility at 6 months
Min, 1994 (60)	IV	Movement return, not blinded	14 patients with unilateral vocal fold paralysis	retrospective analysis	Movement after 6 months
Parnes, 1985 (43)	IV	no	24 patients with vocal fold paralysis	retrospective	Follow-up at 1 year to determine vocal fold movement
Garltan, 1993 (61)	IV	no	4 patients with vocal fold paralysis	case reports	Clinical followup (time not specified)
Gupta, 1993 (62)	IV	no	18 patients with vocal fold paralysis	retrospective	Clinical followup (time not specified)
ElEz, 1998 (44)	IV	no	20 patients with vocal fold paralysis	retrospective	Clinical followup (time not specified
Hirano, 1987 (41)	IV	no	45 patients with complete vocal paralysis	retrospective	Clinical followup (time not specified)

TABLE 4. *Diagnosis of Diseases*

Author Year	Class of Study	Blinded Evaluation	Cohort Size	Comparison Groups	Dx Reference Standard
Schweizer, 1999 (63)	IV	no	2 ALS patients; 1 SD patient post-BOTOX	10 normal controls	no
Yin, 2000 (38)	IV	no	8 patients with neuromuscular disease	11 normal subjects	no

TABLE 5. *Diagnosis of Malingering or*

Author Year	Class of Study	Blinded Evaluation	Cohort Size	Comparison Groups	Dx Reference Standard
None					

Systematic Application of Electrodes and Technique	Measure(s) Used	Sensitivity	Specificity
Bipolar concentric	Classified as neurapraxy or axonotmesis based on opinion of examiner	12.8% accurate prediction of complete recovery	94.4% accurate prediction of poor recovery
Bipolar hooked wires	Duration, amplitude, waveform morphology root-mean-square	89% overall correct prognosis	
Bipolar concentric	Absent or decreased MUP, fibrillation or positive sharp waves	100%	78.6%
Bipolar hooked wires	Presence of sharp waves, MUP	N/A	N/A
"per Hiroto's method"	Presence of voluntary MUP, fibrillations	70% accurate prediction of recovery	75% accurate prediction of poor recovery
"per Hiroto's method"	"Denervation" and interference pattern	55%	100%
bipolar needle	waveform morphology, interference pattern	12/19 (63%) with voluntary MUP recovered	2/10 (20%) with no voluntary MUP recovered motion

Systematic Procedures	Measure(s) Used	Sensitivity	Specificity
yes	Muscle fiber density Jitter mean consecutive fiber difference	Muscle fiber density 66%	Not evaluated
concentric needle EMG	not specified	N/A	N/A

Systematic Procedures	Measure(s) Used	Sensitivity	Specificity

TABLE 6. *Diagnosis of*

Author Year	Class of Study	Blinded Evaluation	Cohort Size	Comparison Groups	Dx Reference Standard
Hillel, 2001 (47)	IV	no	58 patients with SD	10 normal subjects	Clinical assessment, videostrobe
Yin, 2000 (38)	IV	no	24 patients with SD	11 normal subjects	no
Nash, 1996 (64)	IV	no	11 patients with SD	10 normal controls	Videostrobe and speech symptoms
Cyrus, 2001 (65)	IV	no	12 patients with abductor SD	10 normal controls	Videostrobe and speech symptoms

TABLE 7. *Diagnosis of Systemic Neuropathic and*

Author Year	Class of Study	Blinded Evaluation	Cohort Size	Comparison Groups
Dray, 1999 (66)	IV	no	1 patient with Charot-Marie-Tooth disease	case report
Mazzantini, 1998 (67)	IV	no	1 patient with Churg-Strauss	case report

TABLE 8. *Technique for*

Author Year	Class of Study	Blinded Evaluation	Cohort Size	Control Groups
Truong, 1991 (50)	II	double blind	13 patients with adductor SD	yes
Ludlow, 1988 (49)	III	blinded evaluation of speech pre- & post-tx	16 patients with adductor SD	no
Blitzer, 1998 (45)	IV	no	747 patients with adductor/abductor SD	no
Blitzer (46)	IV	no	32 patients with abductor SD	no
Bielamowicz (48)	III	blinded evaluation of speech pre- & post-tx	15 patients with abductor SD	compared endoscopic and percutaneous approaches

Laryngeal Dystonia

Systematic Procedures	Measure(s) Used	Sensitivity	Specificity
monopolar wire EMG	onset latency, amplitude, frequency of muscle activity increased in SD	N/A	N/A
concentric needle EMG	not specified	N/A	N/A
Hooked wire EMG	Mean activity level (percent of max) before and after breaks	N/A	N/A
Hooked wire EMG	Mean activity level (percent of max) before and after breaks	N/A	N/A

Myopathic Disorders Involving the Larynx

Dx Reference Standard	Systematic Procedures	Measure(s) Used	Sensitivity	Specificity
Clinical assessment, extremity EMG	laryngeal EMG (electrode not specified)	MUP morphology, recruitment	N/A	N/A
Clinical assessment, limb EMG, biopsy histology	laryngeal EMG	MUP morphology, recruitment	N/A	N/A

Treatment of Laryngeal Dystonia

Exclusion and Inclusion criteria	Random Assignment	Outcome Measure(s) Used	Accounting for Drop-outs	Baseline Equivalence between Groups
yes	yes	ratings of videotapes and sound spectrograms of sustained vowels; patient self-ratings	no dropouts	no
yes	no	pitch and voice breaks; phonatory aperiodicity, sentence time	no dropouts	N/A
yes	no	subjective rating scale	no	N/A
yes	no	subjective rating scale; Unified SD Rating Scale	no	N/A
yes	crossover design	breathy break counts; patient self-ratings	no	N/A

Although this study provides class II evidence for improvement with botulinum toxin and not saline treatment, laryngeal EMG was used to guide injection with both treatments, so this article does provides class IV evidence on the usefulness of laryngeal EMG over other methods for injection. The usefulness of laryngeal EMG in the treatment of spasmodic dysphonia is also supported by two other studies with class IV evidence.[44,45] Thus, this evidence-based medicine review supports the possible usefulness of laryngeal EMG in the treatment of spasmodic dysphonia.

It has been asserted that laryngeal EMG may be preferable to direct visualization for guidance of botulinum toxin injections for three main reasons. First, using direct visualization requires either sedation/anesthetic in the operating room (direct laryngoscopy) or transoral injection. Many patients find the transoral procedure uncomfortable, and it can only be performed in patients with easily controlled gag reflexes. The use of a flexible injection needle through a bronchoscope is not standard. With this method, precision is difficult to control, and an unacceptable amount of botulinum toxin is wasted because of the length of the flexible, trans-bronchoscopic syringe. Second, when using direct visualization, only the location of the thyroarytenoid can be well visualized. The locations of the lateral cricoarytenoid and posterior cricoarytenoid are more difficult to establish visually. The cricothyroid muscle cannot be seen, although its points of attachment and insertion can be palpated through the neck. Third, laryngeal EMG permits functional confirmation that the needle is in the correct muscle (each muscle has a different electrophysiologic response). It also allows the physician to select the most active part of the muscle, as well as permitting an assessment of the effect of any residual botulinum toxin in patients who are undergoing re-injection. Hence, laryngeal EMG has been considered helpful in facilitating treatment with botulinum toxin.

Class IV evidence also suggests the usefulness of laryngeal EMG in diagnosis and prognosis. A large number of articles suggest that laryngeal EMG is useful in distinguishing vocal fold paresis from mechanical fixation or no abnormality.[3,6,22,39-41,48, 49,51-56,58,59] Seven of these articles suggest that the sensitivity of laryngeal EMG may range from 33% to 100% in detecting vocal fold paresis and that its specificity ranges from 12% to 50%.[6,22,41,52,55,58] Regarding the prognosis of vocal fold paresis, the sensitivity for laryngeal

EMG is predicting recovery ranges from 13% to 100%, whereas the specificity for predicting poor recovery has varied from 20% to 100%.[38,41-44,60-63] Laryngeal EMG may be useful in aiding the identification of muscle activation abnormalities in laryngeal dystonias.[38,47,64,65] Two case reports have suggested that laryngeal EMG was helpful in the diagnosis of a systemic neuropathy.[66,67]

CONCLUSIONS BASED ON REVIEW OF EVIDENCE-BASED DATA

Based on the previously discussed studies, use of laryngeal EMG in the administration of botulinum toxin in the treatment of adductor spasmodic dysphonia is supported by current research at a *Recommendation C* level—possibly useful or predictive for a given condition in the specified population.

RECOMMENDATIONS

Practice recommendations

In the treatment of spasmodic dysphonia, laryngeal EMG localization for the injection of botulinum toxin Type A into the thyroarytenoid muscle for the treatment of adductor spasmodic dysphonia is possibly equal in effectiveness to endoscopic guided injection (Recommendation C).

Recommendations for future research on potential clinical utility of laryngeal electromyography for patients with suspected laryngeal movement disorders

Although evidence-based research is lacking regarding the utility of laryngeal EMG for patients with suspected movement disorders, the large number of studies suggesting its utility[1-36] and its current clinical use indicate the urgent need for a well-controlled study of the accuracy and clinical value of this procedure. The current lack of evidence is because of the absence of high-quality evidence-based research investigating these applications. There is no evidence suggesting that laryngeal EMG is not useful. Research is therefore needed to confirm or refute the clinical value of laryngeal EMG for the other clinical questions investigated.

The studies currently available on this issue include biases and lack standardization in methodology. Few evidence-based studies have investigated the many common clinical uses of laryngeal EMG. Masking (blinding) is a critical feature of the study design that must be included in future studies. To determine the diagnostic or prognostic utility without bias, clinical investigators need to be blinded to patient diagnosis or treatment outcome when interpreting laryngeal EMG findings. For example, representative segments of laryngeal EMG recordings from patients and control subjects could be randomized and interpreted by independent electrodiagnostic medicine consultants at different sites. Random insertion of repeats of some of the individual recordings would permit assessment of intrarater as well as inter-rater reliability for the proposed application. For therapeutic studies, double blinding (masking of both patient or subject and the investigator) should be employed if possible to minimize bias and to allow assessment of placebo effects.

Careful consideration should be given to selection of the best possible "reference standard" by which the presence or absence of a condition is determined for diagnostic or prognostic applications of laryngeal EMG. If the validity of the reference standard in a study is suspect, the validity of the results will be limited accordingly. For applications in which the current reference standard is based on subjective assessments (eg, interpretation of laryngeal endoscopic examinations for the diagnosis of vocal fold paralysis), attempts should be made to define clearly the criteria used for the assessment and consideration should be given to the use of multiple raters to enhance the accuracy of the determination.

In conclusion, additional evidence-based studies are recommended to determine the value of laryngeal EMG for each of the clinical uses for which it is currently being employed, the optimal electrode type for specific clinical purposes, the validity and reliability of techniques used for quantification of laryngeal EMG signals, and the predictive and diagnostic accuracy of EMG findings and their relation to treatment outcomes.

TOOLS

The review of the articles for the evidence-based tables was conducted by reading the articles and recording the results in *Microsoft Excel* (Microsoft Corporation, Redmond, Washington) files under each of the headings provided. No automatic algorithms were used in the procedures.

DISCLAIMER

This report is provided as an educational service of the AAEM, The American Academy of Otolaryngology—Head and Neck Surgery, and The Voice Foundation. It is based on an assessment of the current scientific and clinical information. It is not intended to include all possible methods of care of a particular clinical problem, or all legitimate criteria for choosing to use a specific procedure. Neither is it intended to exclude any reasonable alternative methodologies. This statement is not intended to address all possible uses of, or issues regarding, laryngeal EMG and in no way reflects on the usefulness of laryngeal EMG in those areas not addressed. The AAEM recognizes that specific patient care decisions are the prerogative of the patient and his/her physician and are based on all of the circumstances involved. These guidelines are not a substitute for the experience and judgment of a physician. This review was not written with the intent that it be used as a basis for reimbursement decisions.

REFERENCES

1. Weddel G, Feinstein B, Pattle RE. The electrical activity of voluntary muscle in man under normal and pathological conditions. *Brain.* 1944;67:178–257.
2. Faaborg-Andersen K, Buchtal F. Action potentials from internal laryngeal muscles during phonation. *Nature.* 1956;177:340–341.
3. Faaborg-Andersen K. Electromyographic investigation of intrinsic laryngeal muscles in humans. *Acta Physiol.* 1957;41:1–149.
4. Buchtal F. Electromyography of intrinsic laryngeal muscles. *J Exp Physiol.* 1959;44:137–148.

5. Dedo HH, Hall WN. Electrodes in laryngeal electromyography. Reliability comparison. *Ann Otol Rhinol Laryngol.* 1969;78:172–180.
6. Dedo HH. The paralyzed larynx: an electromyographical study in dogs and humans. *Laryngoscope.* 1970;80:1445–1517.
7. English ET, Blevins CE. Motor units of laryngeal muscles. *Arch Otolaryngol.* 1969;89:778–784.
8. Fex S. Judging the movements of vocal cords in larynx paralysis. *Acta Otolaryngol (Stockh).* 1970;263:82–83.
9. Gay T, Hirose H, Strome M, Sawashima M. Electromyography of the intrinsic laryngeal muscles during phonation. *Ann Otolaryngol.* 1972;81:401–409.
10. Haglund S. Electromyography in the diagnosis of laryngeal motor disorders. Doctoral dissertation, Departments of Otolaryngology and Clinical Neurophysiology, Karolinska Institutet, Stockholm, Sweden, 1973.
11. Haglund S. The normal electromyogram in human cricothyroid muscle. *Acta Otolaryngol (Stockh).* 1973;75:448–453.
12. Haglund S, Knutsson E, Martensson A. An electromyographic study of the vocal and cricothyroid muscles in functional dysphonia. *Acta Otolaryngol (Stockh).* 1974;77:140–149.
13. Hast MH. Mechanical properties of the cricothyroid muscle. *Laryngoscope.* 1966;75:537–548.
14. Hast MH. Mechanical properties of the vocal fold muscles. *Practica Oto-Rhino-Laryngologica.* 1967;33:209–214.
15. Hast MH, Golbus S. Physiology of the lateral cricoarytenoid muscles. *Practica Oto-Rhino-Laryngologica.* 1971;33:209–214.
16. Hirano M, Ohala J. Use of hooked-wire electrodes for electromyography of the intrinsic laryngeal muscles. *J Speech Hear Res.* 1969;12:361–373.
17. Hirano M, Ohala J, Vennard W. The function of laryngeal muscles in regulating fundamental frequency and intensity of phonation. *J Speech Hear Res.* 1969;12:616–628.
18. Hirano M, Vennard W, Ohala J. Regulation of register, pitch and intensity of voice. *Fola Phoniatr.* 1970;22:1–20.
19. Hirose H, Gay T, Strome M. Electrode insertion techniques for laryngeal electromyography. *J Acoust Soc Am.* 1971;50:1449–1450.
20. Hirose H. Clinical observations on 600 cases of recurrent laryngeal nerve palsy. *Annu Bull RILP (Research Institute of Logopedics and Phoniatrics).* 1977;11:165–173.
21. Hiroto I, Hirano M, Toyozumi Y, Shin T. A new method of placement of a needle electrode in the intrinsic laryngeal muscles for electromyography. Insertion through the skin. *Pract Otol (Kyoto).* 1962;55:499–504.

22. Hiroto I, Hirano M, Tomita H. Electromyographic investigation of human vocal cord paralysis. *Ann Otol Rhinol Laryngol.* 1968;77: 296-304.
23. Jonsson B, Reichmann S. Displacement and deformation of wire electrodes in electromyography. *Electromyography.* 1969;9:210-211.
24. Knutsson E, Martensson A, Martensson B. The normal electromyogram in human vocal fold muscles. *Acta Otolaryngol (Stockh).* 1969;68: 526-536.
25. Martensson A, Skoglund CR. Contraction properties of intrinsic laryngeal muscles. *Acta Phys Scand.* 1964;60:318-336.
26. Shipp T, Doherty T, Morrissey P. Predicting vocal frequency from selected physiologic measures. *J Acoust Soc Am.* 1979; 66:678-684.
27. Sussman HM, McNeilage PG, Powers RK. Recruitment and discharge patterns of single motor units during speech production. *J Speech Hear Res.* 1977;20:613-630.
28. Yanagihara N, von Leden H. The cricothyroid muscle during phonation-electromyographic, aerodynamic and acoustic studies. *Ann Otol Rhinol Laryngol.* 1968;75:987-1006.
29. Arnold G. Physiology and pathology of the cricothyroid muscle. *Laryngoscope.* 1961;71:687-753.
30. Hirano M. The function of the intrinsic laryngeal muscles in singing. In: Stevens K, Hirano M, eds. *Vocal Fold Physiology.* Tokyo, Japan: University of Tokyo Press; 1981:155-167.
31. Hirano M. Electromyography of laryngeal muscles. In: Hirano M, ed. *Clinical Examination of Voice.* Wien: Springer Verlag; 1981:11-24.
32. Hirano M. Examination of vocal fold vibration. In: Hirano M, ed. *Clinical Examination of the Voice.* New York: Springer Verlag; 1981:43-65.
33. Hirose H, Kobayashi T, Okamura M, Kurauchi Y, Iwamura S, Uschijima T, et al. Recurrent laryngeal nerve palsy. *J Otolaryngol (Japan).* 1967;70:1-17.
34. Khan A, Pearlman RC, Bianchi DA, Hauck KW. Experience with two types of electromyography monitoring electrodes during thyroid surgery. *Am J Otolaryngol.* 1997;18:99-102.
35. Lindestad PA. *Electromyographic and Laryngoscopic Studies of Normal and Disturbed Voice Function.* Stockholm, Sweden: Departments of Logopedics and Phoniatrics and Clinical Neurophysiology, Huddinge University Hospital; 1994:1-43 and Appendices I-VI.
36. Sataloff RT, Mandel S, Manon-Espaillat R, Heman-Ackah YD, Abaza M. *Laryngeal Electromyography.* Albany, NY: Delmar Thomson Learning; 2003:1-128.
37. Goodin DS, Edlund W. Process for developing technology assessments. American Academy of Neurology Therapeutics and Technology

Assessment Subcommittee, American Academy of Neurology, September 1999, pp. 1–37.

38. Yin S, Qui W, Stucker F, et al. Critical evaluation of neurolaryngological disorders. *Ann Otol Rhinol Laryngol.* 2000;109:832–838.

39. Kokesh J, Flint PW, Robinson LR, Cummings CW. Correlation between stroboscopy and electromyography in laryngeal paralysis. *Ann Otol Rhinol Laryngol.* 1993;102: 852–857.

40. Koufman JA, Postma GN, Whang CS, Rees CJ, Amin MR, Belafsky PC. Diagnostic laryngeal electromyography: the Wake Forest experience 1995–1999. *Otolaryngol Head Neck Surg.* 2001;124:603–606.

41. Hirano M, Nozoe I, Shin T, Maeyama T. Electromyography for laryngeal paralysis. In: Hirano M, Kirchner JA, Bless DM, eds. *Neurolaryngology: Recent Advances.* Boston, MA: College-Hill Press; 1987:232–248.

42. Sittel C, Stennert E, Thumfart WF, Dapunt V, Eckel HE. Prognostic value of laryngeal electromyography in vocal fold paralysis. *Arch OtolaryngolHead Neck Surg.* 2001;127:155–160.

43. Parnes SM, Satya-Murti S. Predictive value of laryngeal electromyography in patients with vocal cord paralysis of neurogenic origin. *Laryngoscope.* 1985;95:1323–1326.

44. Elez F, Celik M. The value of laryngeal electromyography in vocal cord paralysis [letter]. *Muscle Nerve.* 1998;21:552–553.

45. Blitzer A, Brin MF, Stewart CF. Botulinum toxin management of spasmodic dysphonia (laryngeal dystonia): a 12-year experience in more than 900 patients. *Laryngoscope.* 1998;108:1435–1441.

46. Blitzer A, Brin MF, Stweart C, Aviv JE, Fahn S. Abductor laryngeal dystonia: a series treated with botulinum toxin. *Laryngoscope.* 1992;102:163–167.

47. Hillel AD. The study of laryngeal muscle activity in normal human subjects and in patients with laryngeal dystonia using multiple fine-wire electromyography. *Laryngoscope.* 2001;111(4 part 2 Suppl 97):1–47.

48. Bielamowicz S, Squire S, Bidus K, Ludlow C. Assessment of posterior cricoarytenoid botulinum toxin injections in patients with abductor spasmodic dysphonia. *Ann Otol Rhinol Laryngol.* 2001;110:406–412.

49. Ludlow CL, Naunton RF, Sedory SE, Schulz GM, Hallett M. Effects of botulinum toxin injections on speech in adductor spasmodic dysphonia. *Neurology.* 1988;38:1220–1225.

50. Truong DD, Rontal M, Rolnick M, Aronson AE, Mistura K. Double-blind controlled study of botulinum toxin in adductor spasmodic dysphonia. *Laryngoscope.* 1991;101:630–634.

51. Satoh I. Evoked electromyographic test applied for recurrent laryngeal nerve paralysis. *Laryngoscope.* 1978;88:2022–2031.

52. Haglund S, Knutsson E, Martensson A. An electromyographic analysis of idiopathic vocal cord paresis. *Acta Otolaryngol.* 1972;74:265–270.

53. Rontal E, Rontal M, Silverman B, Kileny PR. The clinical differentiation between vocal cord paralysis and vocal cord fixation using electromyography. *Laryngoscope.* 1993;103:133–137.

54. Miller RH, Rosenfield DB. The role of electromyography in clinical laryngology. *Otolaryngol Head Neck Surg.* 1984;92:287–291.

55. Lindestad PA, Persson A. Quantitative analysis of EMG interference pattern in patients with laryngeal paresis. *Acta Otolaryngol.* 1994; 114:91–97.

56. Dray TG, Robinson LR, Hillel AD. Idiopathic bilateral vocal fold weakness. *Laryngoscope.* 1999;109:995–1002.

57. Yin SS, Qiu WW, Stucker FJ. Major patterns of laryngeal electromyography and their clinical application. *Laryngoscope.* 1997;107: 126–136.

58. Blair RL, Berry H, Briant TD. Laryngeal electromyography—techniques, applications, and a review of personal experience. *J Otolaryngol.* 1977;6:496–504.

59. Haglund S, Knutsson E, Martensson A. Neurogenic lesions in the cricothyroid muscle in idiopathic vocal cord paresis. *Acta Otolaryngol.* 1973;76(1):63–69.

60. Min YB, Finnegan EMG, Hoffman HT, Luscheri ES, McCulloch TM. A preliminary study of the prognostic role of electromyography in laryngeal paralysis. *Otolaryngol Head Neck Surg.* 1994;111:770–775.

61. Gartlan MG, Hoffman HT. Crystalline preparation of botulinum toxin type A (Botox): degradation in potency with storage. *Otolaryngol Head Neck Surg.* 1993;108:135–140.

62. Gupta SR, Bastian RW. Use of laryngeal electromyography in prediction of recovery after vocal cord paralysis [letter]. *Muscle Nerve.* 1993; 16:977–978.

63. Schweizer V, Woodson GE, Bertorini TE. Single-fiber electromyography of the laryngeal muscles. *Muscle Nerve.* 1999;22:111–114.

64. Nash EA, Ludlow CL. Laryngeal muscle activity during speech breaks in adductor spasmodic dysphonia. *Laryngoscope.* 1996;106:484–489.

65. Cyrus CB, Bielamowicz S, Evans FJ, Ludlow CL. Adductor muscle activity abnormalities in abductor spasmodic dysphonia. *Otolarynogl Head Neck Surg.* 2001;124:23–30.

66. Dray TG, Robinson LR, Hillel AD. Laryngeal electromyographic findings in Charcot-Marie-Tooth disease type II. *Arch Neurol.* 1999;56: 863–865.

67. Mazzantini M, Fattori B, Mattrucci F, Gaeta P, Ursino F. Neuro-laryngeal involvement in Churg-Strauss syndrome. *Eur Arch Otorhinolaryngol.* 1998;255:302–306.

APPENDIX III

Suggested Reading

Abaza M, Sataloff RT, Hawkshaw MJ, Mandel S. Laryngeal manifestations of post poliomyelitis syndrome. *J Voice.* 2001;14(3):291–294.

Adams SG, Hunt EJ, Charles DA, Lang AE. Unilateral versus bilateral botulinum toxin injections in spasmodic dysphonia: acoustic and perceptual results. *J Otolaryngology.* 1993;22(3):171–175.

Allen CD, Bernstein B, Chait DH. EMG biofeedback treatment of pediatric hyperfunctional dysphonia. *J Behav Ther & Exp Psychiatry.* 1991; 22(2):97–101.

Aminoff MJ. Properties and functional organization of motor units. In: Aminoff, MJ. *Electromyography in Clinical Practice.* 3rd ed. New York, NY: Churchill Livingston; 1998:33.

Aminoff MJ. Clinical electromyography. In: Aminoff MJ, ed. Electrodiagnosis in *Clinical Neurology.* 4th ed. Philadelphia, Pa: Churchill Livingston; 1999: 223–252.

Andreassen S. Methods for computer-aided measurement of motor unit parameters. *Electroencephalogr Clin Neurophysiol Suppl.* 1987;39: 13–20.

Andrews S, Warner J, Stewart R. EMG biofeedback and relaxation in the treatment of hyperfunctional dysphonia. *Br J Disord Commun.* 1986; 21(3):353–369.

Arnold G. Physiology and pathology of the cricothyroid muscle. *Laryngoscope.* 1961;71:687–753.

Arold R, Limberg C. Electromyography of the larynx. *HNO.* 1983;31(10): 353–358.

Arunodava FR, Shenoy AM, Premalata S. Electromyography in near-total laryngectomy. *Arch Otolaryngol Head Neck Surg.* 1998;124(8):857–860.

Atkinson SI, Rees J. Botulinum toxin for endopharyngeal dysphagia: case reports of CT-guided injection. *J Otolaryngol.* 1997;26(4):273–276.

Basmajian JV, Stecko G. A new bipolar electrode for electromyography. *J Appl Physiol.* 1962;17:849.

Bennett JD, Chowdhury CR. Primary amyloidosis of the larynx. *J Laryngol Otol.* 1994;108:339–340.

Benninger MS, Gillen JB, Altman JS. Changing etiology of vocal fold immobility. *Laryngoscope.* 1998;108(9):1346–1350.

Berg AM, Troxler RF, Grillone G, Kasznica J, Kane K, Cohen AS, Skinner M. Localized amyloidosis of the larynx: evidence for light chain composition. *Ann Otol Rhinol Laryngol.* 1993;102:884–889.

Bergmans J. Computer assisted on line measurement of motor unit parameters in human electromyography. *Electromyography.* 1971;11: 161–181.

Berkowitz, RG. Laryngeal electromyography findings in idiopathic congenital bilateral vocal cord paralysis. *Ann Otol Rhinol Laryngol.* 1996; 105(3):207–212.

Bertorini TE, Stalberg E, Yuson CP, et al. Single fiber electromyography in neuromuscular disorders: correlation of muscle histochemistry, single-fiber electromyography, and clinical findings. *Muscle Nerve.* 1994; 17:345–353.

Bischoff C, Stalberg E, Flack B, et al: Reference values of motor unit action potentials obtained with multi-MUAP analysis. *Muscle Nerve.* 1994; 17:842–851.

Blitzer A. Laryngeal electromyography. In: Rubin J, Sataloff RT, Korovin G, Gould W., eds. *Diagnosis and Treatment of Voice Disorders.* New York, NY: Igaku-Shoin Ltd.; 1995:316–326.

Blitzer A, Brin M, Fahn S, Lovelace RE. Clinical and laboratory characteristics of focal laryngeal dystonia: study of 110 cases. *Laryngoscope.* 1988;98: 636–640.

Blitzer A, Brin M, Sasaki C. *Neurological Disorders of the Larynx.* New York, NY: Theime, 1992.

Blitzer A, Brin MF, Stewart C, Aviv JE, Fahn S. Abductor laryngeal dystonia; a series treated with botulinum toxin. *Laryngoscope.* 1992;102(2): 163-167.

Blitzer A, Jahn AF, Keidar A. Semon's law revisited: an electromyographic analysis of laryngeal synkinesis. *Ann Otol Rhinol Laryngol.* 1996; 105(10): 764-769.

Blitzer A, Lovelace RE, Brin MF, Fahn S, Fink ME. Electromyographic findings in focal laryngeal dystonia (spasmodic dysphonia). *Ann Otol Rhinol Laryngol.* 1985;94:591-594.

Boemke W, Gerull G, Hippel K. Electromyography of the larynx with skin surface electrodes. *Folia Phoniatr (Basel).* 1992;44(5):220-230.

Bradley WG, Tandan R. Dermatomyositis and polymuyositis. In: Wilson JD, Braunwald E, Isselbacher KJ, Petersdorf RG, Martin JB Fauci AS, Root RK, eds. *Harrison's Principles of Internal Medicine.* 12th ed. New York, NY: McGraw-Hill, Inc.; 1991:2108-2111.

Brancatisano A, Dodd DS, Engel LA. Posterior cricoarytenoid activity and glottic size during hyperpnea in humans. *J Appl Physiol.* 1991; 71(3): 977-982.

Brandstater ME, Lambert EH. Motor unit anatomy. type and spatial arrangement of muscle fibers. In: Desmedt JE, ed. *New Developments in Electromyography and Clinical Neurophysiology.* Basel, Switzerland: Karger; 1971:14-22.

Bridger MW, Jahn AF, van Vostrand AW. Laryngeal rheumatoid arthritis. *Laryngoscope.* 1980; 90:296-303.

Bromberg MB, Forshaw DA, Nau HL, et al. Motor unit number estimation, isometric strength and electromyography measures in amyotrophic lateral sclerosis. *Muscle Nerve.* 1993;16:1213-1219.

Bromberg MB, Scott DM, Ad Hoc Committee of the AAEM Special Interest Single Fiber EMG Group. Single fiber EMG reference values: reformatted in tabular form. *Muscle Nerve.* 1994;17(7):820-821.

Broniatowski M, Grundfest-Broniatowski S, Davies CR, Jacobs GB, Tucker HM, Nose Y. Electronic pacing of incapacitated head and neck structures. *ASAIO Transactions.* 1991;37(4):553-558.

Brooke MH, Engle WK. The histographic analysis of human muscle biopsies with regard to fibre types. 1. Adult male and female. *Neurology.* 1969;19: 221-233.

Brown WF. A method for estimating the number of motor units in thenar muscles and the changes in motor unit count with aging. *J Neurol Neurosurg Psychiatry.* 1972;35:845-852.

Brown WF. *The Physiological and Technical Basis of Electromyography.* Stoneham, Mass: Butterworth Publishers; 1984.

Brown WF, Milner-Brown HS. Some electrical properties of motor units and their effects on the methods of estimating motor unit numbers. *J Neurol Neurosurg Psychiatry.* 1976;39:249-368.

Brown WF, Strong MJ, Smow R. Methods for estimating numbers of motor units in biceps-brachialis muscles and losses of motor units with aging. *Muscle Nerve.* 1988;11:423-432.

Buchtal F. *An Introduction to Electromyography.* Copenhagen: Scandinavian University Books; 1957.

Buchtal F. Electromyography of intrinsic laryngeal muscles. *J Exp Physiol.* 1959;44:137-148.

Buchtal F, Guld C, Rosenfalck P. Action potential parameters in normal human muscle and their dependence on physical variables. *Acta Physiol Scand.* 1954;32:200-218.

Buchtal F, Kamienciecka Z. The diagnostic yield of quantified electromyography and quantified muscle biopsy in neuromuscular disorders. *Muscle Nerve.* 1982;5:265-280.

Buchtal F, Pinelli P, Rosenfalck P. Action potential parameters in normal human muscle and their physiological determinants. *Acta Physiol Scand.* 1954;32:219-229.

Burke RE. Physiology of motor unit. In: Engle AG, Franzini-Armstrong C, eds. *Myology.* New York, NY: McGraw-Hill; 1994:164.

Campbell WW. Needle electrode examination. In: Campbell WW, ed. *Essentials of Neurodiagnostic Medicine.* Baltimore, Md: Williams & Wilkins; 1999:93-116.

Campbell MJ, McComas AJ, Petito F. Physiological changes in aging muscles. *J Neurol Neurosurg Psychiatry.* 1973;36:174-182.

Canals Ruiz P, Villoslada Prieto C, Lopez Catala F, Peris Beaufils JL, Marco Peiro A, Marco Algarra J. Standard electromyography for the diagnosis and prognosis of laryngeal neuromuscular disorders. *Acta Otorrinolaringol Esp.* 1995;46(3):203-207.

Cao J, Sander DB. Multivariate discriminant analysis of the electromyographic interference pattern: A statistical approach to discrimination among controls, myopathies and neuropathies. *Med Biol Eng Comput.* 1996;34:369-374.

Chanaud CM, Ludlow CL. Single motor unit activity of human intrinsic laryngeal muscles during respiration. *Ann Otol Rhinol Laryngol.* 1992;101(10):832-840.

Clark WD. Diagnosis and stating of laryngeal disease. In: Bailey BJ, Biller HJ, eds. *Non-serial; Surgery of the Larynx.* Philadelphia, Pa: W.B. Saunders Company; 1985:45-52

Clayman D, Booth RP, Isaacs J Jr, Russo LS Jr. Percutaneous electromyography of the posterior cricoarytenoid muscles: electromyographic needle placement with computed tomographic guidance. *Laryngoscope.* 1994;1004(11 pt 1):1393–1396.

Cohen AS. Amyloidosis. In: Wilson JD, Braunwald E, Isselbacher KJ, Petersdorf RG, Martin JB Fauci AS, Root RK, eds. *Harrison's principles of internal medicine.* 12th ed. New York, NY: McGraw-Hill, Inc.; 1991: 1417–1421.

Crevier-Buchman L, Laccourreve O, Papon JF, Nurit D, Brasnu D. Adductor spasmodic dysphonia: case reports with acoustic analysis following botulinum toxin injection and acupuncture. *J Voice.* 1997;11(2): 232–237.

Crumley RL. Laryngeal synkinesis: its significance to the laryngologist. *Ann Otol Rhinol Laryngol.* 1989;98(2):87–92.

Crumley RL, Horn K, Clendenning D. Laryngeal reinnervation using the split-phrenic nerve-graft procedure. 1980;88(2):159–164.

Daniels SK, Mahoney MC, Lyons GD. Persistent dysphagia and dysphonia following cervical spine surgery. *Ear Nose Throat J.* 1998;77(6):473–475.

Dantes M, McComas A. The extent and time course of motorneuron involvement in amyotrophic lateral sclerosis. *Muscle Nerve.* 1991;14: 416–421.

Daube JR. Statistical estimates of number of motor units in the thenar and foot muscles in patients with amyotrophic lateral sclerosis or the residual of poliomyelitis. *Muscle Nerve.* 1988;11:957–958.

Daube JR. AAEM minimonograph #11: needle examination in clinical electromyography. *AAEM.* 1991;1–23.

Daube JR. Estimating the number of motor units in a muscle. *J Clin Neurophysiol.* 1995;12:585–594.

Daube JR. Assessing the motor unit with needle electromyography. In: Daube JR, ed. *Clinical Neurophysiology.* Philadelphia, Pa: Davis; 1996:257–281.

Davidson BJ, Ludlow, CL. Long-term effects of botulinum toxin injections in spasmodic dysphonia. *Ann Otol Rhinol Laryngol.* 1996;105(1): 33–42.

de Koning P, Wieneke GH, vad der Most, van Spijk D, et al. Estimation of the number of motor units based on macro-EMG. *J Neurol Neurosurg Psychiatry.* 1988;51:403–411.

de Oliveira JT, Levy-Reis I. Syndrome of continuous muscle fiber activity. case report 11-year follow-up. *Arquivos de Neuro-Psiquiatria.* 1994; 52(1):96–99.

Dedo HH. The paralyzed larynx: an electromyographical study in dogs and humans. *Laryngoscope.* 1970;80:1445–1517.

Dedo HH, Hall WN. Electrodes in laryngeal electromyography. reliability comparison. *Ann Otol Rhinol Laryngol.* 1969;78:172–180.

Dejonckere P, Hamoir M. Etiology of neurogenic laryngeal lesions diagnosed by electromyography. *Acta Otorhinolaryngol Belg.* 1980;34(3): 285-299.

Dengler R, Konstanzer A, Kuther G, et al. Amyotrophic lateral sclerosis: macro-EMG and twitch forces of single motor units. *Muscle Nerve.* 1990;13:545-550.

Desmedt JE, Borenstein S. Relationship of spontaneous fibrillation potentials of muscle fibre segmentation in human muscular dystrophy. *Nature.* 1975;258:531-534.

Dhonneur G, Kirov K, Slavov V, Duvaldestin P. Effects of an intubating dose of succinylcholine and rocuronium on the larynx and diaphragm: an electromyographic study in humans. *Anesthesiology.* 1999;90(4):951-955.

Doherty TJ, Brown WF. The estimated numbers and relative sizes of thenar motor units as selected by multiple point stimulation in young and older adults. *Muscle Nerve.* 1993;16:355-365.

Doherty TJ, Komori T, Stashuk DW, et al. Physiological properties of single thenar motor units in the F-response of younger and older adults. *Muscle Nerve.* 1994;17:860-872.

Doherty T, Simmons Z, O'Connell B, et al. Methods for estimating the numbers of motor units in human muscles. *J Clin Neurophysiol.* 1994; 12:565-584.

Doherty TJ, Stashuk DW, Brown WF. Determinants of mean motor unit size: impact on estimates of motor unit number. *Muscle Nerve.* 1993;16: 1326-1331.

Doherty TJ, Vandervoort AA, Brown WF. Effects of ageing on the motor unit: a brief review. *Can J Appl Physiol.* 1993;19:331-358.

Dorfman L, Howard J, McGill K. Clinical studies using automatic decomposition electromyography (ADEMG) in needle and surface EMG. In: Desmedt JE, ed. *Computer Aided Electromyography and Expert Systems. Clinical Neurophysiology Updates.* Amsterdam: Elsevier; 1989:189-204.

Dorfman LJ, McGill KC. AAEE minimonograph #29: automatic quantitative electromyography. *Muscle Nerve.* 1988;11:804-818.

Dray TG, Robinson LR, Hillel AD. Idiopathic bilateral vocal fold weakness. *Laryngoscope.* 1999;109:995-1002.

Dray TG, Robinson LR, Hillel AD. Laryngeal electromyographic findings in Charcot-Marie-Tooth disease type II. *Arch Neurol.* 1999;56:863-865.

Driscoll BP, Gracco C, Coelho C, et al. Laryngeal function in postpolio patients. *Laryngoscope.* 1995;105(1):35-41.

Dubowit CV, Pearse AGE. A comparative histochemical study of oxidative enzyme and phosphorylase activity in skeletal muscles. *Histochemie.* 1960;2:105.

Dursun G, Sataloff RT, Spiegel JR, Mandel S, Heuer RJ, Rosen DC. Superior laryngeal nerve paresis and paralysis. *J Voice.* 1996;10(2):206-211.

Dyhr H. The activity of the cricothyroid muscle and the intrinsic fundamental frequency in Danish vowels. *Phonetica.* 1990;47(3-4):141-154.

Eckel HE, Sittel C. Morphometry of the larynx in horizontal sections. *Am J Otolaryngol.* 1995;16(1):40-48.

Eckel HE, Sittel C, Zorowka P, Jerke A. Dimensions of the laryngeal framework in adults. *Surg Radiol Anat.* 1994;16(1):31-36.

Eckley CA, Sataloff RT, Hawkshaw M, Spiegel JR, Mandel S. Voice range in superior laryngeal nerve paresis and paralysis. *J Voice.* 1998;12(3): 340-348.

Efendiev AE, Kutukov IuN, Redenko DI. Electromyography in the evaluation of the functional state of the internal neuromuscular apparatus of the larynx in myasthenia. *Vestn Otorinolaringol.* 1991;(6):21-24.

Eger CE, Huxtable CR, Chester ZC, Summers BA. Progressive tetraparesis and laryngeal paralysis in a young rottweiler with neuronal vacuolation and axonal degeneration: an Australian case. *Aust Vest J.* 1998; 76(11):733-737.

Eichenwald EC, Howell RG 3rd, Kosch PC, Ungarelli RA, Lindsey J, Stark R. Developmental changes in sequential activation of laryngeal abductor muscles and diaphragm in infants. *J Appl Physiol.* 1992;73(4): 1425-1431.

Eichenwald EC, Ungarelli RA, Stark AR. Hypercapnia increases expiratory braking in preterm infants. *J Appl Physiol.* 1993;75(6):2665-2670.

Ekstedt J. Human single muscle fibre action potentials. *Acta Physiol Scand.* 1964, (suppl. 226):1-96.

Ekstedt J, Stalberg E. A method of recording extracellular action potentials of single muscle fibres and measuring their propagation velocity in voluntarily activated human muscle. *Bull Am Assoc EMG Electrodiagn.* 1963;10:16.

Ekstedt J, Stalberg E. Abnormal connections between skeletal muscle fibers. *Electroencephalogr Clin Neurophysiol.* 1969;27:607-609.

Ekstedt J, Stalber E. Single fibre electromyography for the study of the microphysiology of the human muscle. In: Desmedt JE, ed. *New Developments in Electromyography and Clinical Neurophysiology.* Basel: Karger; 1971:89-112.

Ekstedt J, Stalberg E. How the size of the needle electrode leading-off surface influences the shape of the single muscle fibre action potential in electromyography. *Comput Programs Biomed.* 1973;3:204-212.

Ekstedt J, Stalberg E. Single muscle fibre electromyography in myasthenia gravis. In: Kunze K, Desmedt JE, eds. *Studies in Neuromuscular Diseases.* Basel: Karger; 1975:157-161.

Ekstedt J, Nilsson G, Stalberg E. Calculation of the electromyographic jitter. *J Neurosurg Psychiatry.* 1974;37:526-539.

Elez F, Celik M. The value of laryngeal electromyography in vocal cord paralysis [letter]. *Muscle Nerve.* 1998;214(4):552-553.

Engle AG, Labbert EH, Santa T. Study of long-term anticholinesterase therapy. effects on neuromuscular transmission on motor end plate fine structure. *Neurology.* 1973;23:1273-1281.

English ET, Blevins CE. Motor units of laryngeal muscles. *Arch Otolaryngol.* 1969;89:778-784.

Ertekin C, Avdogdu I, Yucevar N, et al. Effects of bolus volume on oropharyngeal swallowing: an electrophysiologic study in man. *Am J Gastroenterology.* 1997;92(11):2049-2053.

Ertekin C, Pehlivan M, Aydogdu I, et al. An electrophysiological investigation of deglutition in man. *Muscle Nerve.* 1995;18(10):1177-1186.

Faaborg-Andersen K. Electromyographic investigation of intrinsic laryngeal muscles in humans. *Acta Physiol.* 1957;41(suppl 140):1-149.

Faaborg-Andersen K, Buchtal F. Action potentials from internal laryngeal muscles during phonation. *Nature.* 1956;177:340-341.

Felice KJ. A longitudinal study comparing thenar motor unit number estimates to other quantitative tests in patients with amyotrophic lateral sclerosis. *Muscle Nerve.* 1997;20:179-185.

Feve A, Angelard B, Fenelon G, Logak M, Guillard A, Lacau Saint-Guily J. Postneuroleptic laryngeal dyskinesias: a cause of upper airway obstructive syndrome improved by local injections of botulinum toxin. *Movement Disorders.* 1993;8(2):217-219.

Fex S. Judging the movements of vocal cords in larynx paralysis. *Acta Otolaryngol (Stockh).* 1970;263:82-83.

Ford, CN. Laryngeal EMG in clinical neurolaryngology [comment]. *Arch Otolaryngol Head Neck Surg.* 1998;124(4):476-477.

Fritzell B, Hammarberg B, Schiratzki H, Haglund S, Knutsson E, Martensson A. Long term results of recurrent laryngeal nerve resection for adductor spasmodic dysphonia. *J Voice.* 1993;7(2):172-178.

Fuglsang-Frederiksen A. Quantitative electromyography-II. modifications of the turns analysis. *Electromyogr Clin Neurophysiol.* 1987;27:335-338.

Fuglsang-Frederiksen A, Dahl K, Lo Monaco M. Electrical muscle activity during a gradual increase in force in patients with neuromuscular disease. *Electroencephalogr Clin Neurophysiol.* 1984;57:320-329.

Fuglsang-Frederiksen A, Lo Monaco M, Dahl K. Turns analysis (peak ratio) in EMG using mean amplitude as a substitute of force measurement. *Electroencephalogr Clin Neurophysiol.* 1985;60:225-227.

Fuglsang-Frederiksen A, Mansson A. Analysis of electrical activity of normal muscle in man at different degrees of voluntary effort. *J. Neurol Neurosurg Psychiatry.* 1975;38:683–694.

Fuglsang-Frederiksen A, Ronager J. EMG power spectrum, turns-amplitude analysis and motor unit potential duration in neuromuscular disorders. *J Neurol Sci.* 1990;97:81–91.

Fuglsang-Frederiksen A, Scheel U, Buchthal F. Diagnostic yield of analysis of the pattern of electrical activity and of individual motor unit potentials in myopathy. *J Neurosurg Psychiatry.* 1976;39:742–750.

Fuglsang-Frederiksen A, Scheel U, Buchtal F. Diagnostic yield of the analysis of the pattern of electrical activity of muscle and of individual motor unit potentials in neurogenic involvement. *J Neurol Neurosurg Psychiatry.* 1977;40:544–554.

Fujita M, Ludlow CL, Woodson GE. A new surface electrode for recording from the posterior cricoarytenoid muscle. *Laryngoscope.* 1989;99: 316–320.

Gabriel P, Chilla R. Indications and timing of conservative surgery of peripheral neurogenic vocal cord paresis (author's trans). *HNO.* 1975; 23(11): 333–336.

Galea V, deBruin H, Cacasin R, et al. The numbers and relative sizes of motor units estimated by computer. *Muscle Nerve.* 1991;14:1123–1130.

Gallivan GJ, Hoffman L, Gallivan KH. Episodic paroxysmal laryngospasm: voice and pulmonary function assessment and management. *J Voice.* 1996;10(1): 93–105.

Gans C, Clark B. Studies on ventilation of Caiman crocodilus (Crocodilia: Reptilia). *Respir Physiol.* 1976;26(3):285–301.

Gartlan MG, Hoffman HT. Crystalline preparation of botulinum of toxin type A (Botox): degradation in potency with storage. *Otolaryngol Head Neck Surg.* 1993;108:135–140.

Gartlan MG, Peterson KL, Luschei ES, Hoffman HT, Smith RJ. Bipolar hooked-wire electromyographic technique in the evaluation of pediatric vocal cord paralysis. *Ann Otol Rhinol Laryngol.* 1993;102(9): 695–700.

Garrett JD, Larson CR. Neurology of the laryngeal system. In: Ford CN, Bless DM, eds. *Phonosurgery.* New York, NY: Raven Press; 1991: 43–76.

Gath I, Stalberg E. On the measurement of fibre density in human muscle. *Electroencephalogr Clin Neurophysiol.* 1982;54:699–706.

Gay T, Hirose H, Strome M, Sawashima M. Electromyography of the intrinsic laryngeal muscles during phonation. *Ann Otolaryngol.* 1972;81: 401–409.

Gay T, Rendell JK, Spiro J. Oral and laryngeal muscle coordination during swallowing. *Laryngoscope.* 1994;104(3 pt 1):341–349.

Gilchrist JM, Ad Hoc Committee of the AAEM Special Interest Group on Single Fiber EMG. Single fiber EMG reference values: a collaborative effort. *Muscle Nerve.* 1992;15:151–161.

Gilchrist JM, Nandedkar SD, Stewart CS, et al. Automatic analysis of the electromyographic interference pattern using the turns/amplitude ratio. *Electroencephalogr Clin Neurophysiol.* 1988;70:534–540.

Gitter AG, Stolov WG. Instrumentation and measurement in electrodiagnostic medicine, part 1. *Muscle Nerve.* 1995;18:799.

Goodman M, Montgomery W, Minette L. Pathologic findings in gouty cricoarytenoid arthritis. *Arch Otolaryngol.* 1976; 102:27–29.

Gould WJ, Kamura H. Static lung volumes in singers. *Ann Otol Rhinol Laryngol.* 1973;82:89–95.

Green CD, Berke GS, Ward PH, Gerratt BR. Point-touch technique of botulinum toxin injection for the treatment of spasmodic dysphonia. *Ann Otol Rhinol Laryngol.* 1992;101(11):883–887.

Grossman A, Martin JR, Root HS. Rheumatoid arthritis of the cricoarytenoid joint. *Laryngoscope.* 1961; 71:530–544.

Grundfast KM, Harley E. Vocal cord paralysis. *Otolaryngol Clin North Am.* 1989;22(3):569–597.

Guindi GM, Bannister R, Gibson WP, Payne JK. Laryngeal electomyography in multiple system atrophy with autonomic failure. *J Neurol Neurosurg Psychiatry.* 1981;44:49–53.

Guindi GM, Higenbottam TW, Payne JK. A new method for laryngeal electromyography. *Clin Otolaryngol.* 1981;6:271–278.

Guld C, Rosenfalck A, Willison RG. Report of the committee on EMG instrumentation, technical factors in recording electrical activity of muscles and nerves in men. *Electroencephalogr, Clin Neurophysiol.* 1970; 28:399.

Gupta SR, Bastian RW. Use of laryngeal electromyography in prediction of recovery after vocal cord paralysis [letter]. *Muscle Nerve.* 1993;16(9): 977–978.

Hagg GM. Interpretation of EMG spectral alterations and alteration indexes at sustained contraction. *J Appl Physiol.* 1992;73:1211–1217.

Haglund S. *Electromyography in the Diagnosis of Laryngeal Motor Disorders* [doctoral dissertation]. Stockholm, Sweden: Karolinska Institutet, Departments of Otolaryngology and Clinical Neurophysiology; 1973.

Haglund S. The normal electromyogram in human cricothyroid muscle. *Acta Otolaryngol (Stockh).* 1973;75:478–453.

Haglund S, Knutsson E, Martensson A. An electromyographic analysis of idiopathic vocal cord paresis. *Acta Otolaryngol.* 1972;74(4):265–270.

Haglund S, Knutsson E, Martensson A. An electromyographic study of the vocal and cricothyroid muscles in functional dysphonia. *Acta Otolaryngol (Stockh).* 1974;77:140–149.

Hakelius L, Stalberg E. Electromyographical studies of free autogenous muscle transplants in man. *Scand J Plast Reconstr Surg.* 1974;8: 211–219.

Hast MH. Mechanical properties of the cricothyroid muscle. *Laryngoscope.* 1966;75:537–548.

Hast MH. Mechanical properties of the vocal fold muscles. *Practica Oto-Rhino-Laryngologica.* 1967;33:209–214.

Hast MH, Golbus S. Physiology of the lateral cricoarytenoid muscles. *Practica Oto-Rhino-Laryngologica.* 1971;33:209–214.

Hayward M. Automatic analysis of the electromyogram in healthy subjects of different ages. *J Neurol Sci.* 1977;33:397–413.

Hayward M, Willison RG. Automatic analysis of the electromyogram in patients with chronic partial denervation. *J Neurol Sci.* 1977;33: 415–423.

Hellquist H, Olofsson J, Sokjer H, Odkvist LM. Amyloidosis of the larynx. *Acta Otolaryngol (Stockh).* 1979;88:443–450.

Henneman E, Clamann HP, Gillies JD, et al. Rank order of motoneurons within a pool: law of combination. *J Neurophysiol.* 1974;37:1338–1349.

Henriksson KG, Stalberg E. The terminal innervation pattern in polymyositis: a histochemical and SFEMG study. *Muscle Nerve.* 1978;1:3–13.

Hertrich I, Lutzenberger W, Spieker S, Ackermann H. Fractal dimension of sustained vowel productions in neurological dysphonias: an acoustic and electroglottographic analysis [letter]. *J Acoust Soc Am.* 1997; 102(1):652–654.

Heuer RJ, Sataloff RT, Emerich K, Rulnick R, Baroody M, Spiegel JR, Dursun G, Butler J. Unilateral recurrent laryngeal nerve paralysis: the importance of "preoperative" voice therapy. *J Voice.* 1997;11(1):88–94.

Hillel AD, Robinson LR, Waugh P. Laryngeal electromyography for the diagnosis and management of swallowing disorders. *Otolaryngol Head Neck Surg.* 1997;116(3):344–348.

Hilton-Brown P, Nandedkar SED, Stalberg EV. Simulation of fibre density in single-fiber electromyography and its relationship to macro-EMG. *Med Biol Eng Comput.* 1985;23:541–546.

Hilton-Brown P, Stalberg E. The motor unit in muscular dystrophy, a single fibre EMG and scanning EMG study. *J Neurol Neurosurg Psychiatry.* 1983;46: 981–995.

Hilton-Brown P, Stalberg E. Motor unit size in muscular dystrophy, a macro EMG and scanning EMG study. *J Neurol Neurosurg Psychiatry.* 1983; 46:996–1005.

Hilton-Brown P, Stalberg EV, Osterman PO. Signs of reinnervation in myasthenia gravis. *Muscle Nerve.* 1982;5:215–221.

Hirano M. Phonosurgery. basic and clinical investigations. *Otologia (Fukuoka).* 1975;21:239–442.

Hirano M. Electomyography of laryngeal muscles. In: Hirano M, ed. *Clinical Examination of Voice.* Wein-New York: Springer-Verlag; 1981: 11–24.

Hirano M. Examination of vocal fold vibration. In: Hirano M. *Clinical Examination of the Voice.* Wien-New York: Springer-Verlag; 1981: 43–65.

Hirano M. The function of the intrinsic laryngeal muscles in singing. In: Stevens K, Hirano M, eds. *Vocal Fold Physiol.* Tokyo, Japan: University of Tokyo Press; 1981:155–167.

Hirano M, Nosoe I, Shin T, Maeyama T. Electromyography for laryngeal paralysis. In: Hirano M, Kirchner J, Bless D, eds. *Neurolaryngology: Recent Advances.* Boston, Mass: College Hill; 1987:232–248.

Hirano M, Ohala J. Use of hooked-wire electrodes for electromyography of the intrinsic laryngeal muscles. *J Speech Hear Res.* 1969;12:361–373.

Hirano M, Ohala J, Vennard W. The function of laryngeal muscles in regulating fundamental frequency and intensity of phonation. *J Speech Hear Res.* 1969;12:616–628.

Hirano M, Tanaka S, Fujita M, Fujita H. Vocal cord paralysis caused by esophageal cancer surgery. *Ann Otol Rhinol Laryngol.* 1993;102(3 pt 1): 182–185.

Hirano M, Vennard W, Ohala J. Regulation of register, pitch and intensity of voice. *Folia Phoniatr.* 1970;22:1–20.

Hirose H. Clinical observations on 600 cases of recurrent laryngeal nerve palsy. *Annual Bull RILP* (Research Institute of Logopedics and Phoniatrics), University of Tokyo 1977;11:165–173.

Hirose H, Gay T, Strome M. Electrode insertion techniques for laryngeal electromyography. *J Acoust Soc Am.* 1971;50:1449–1450.

Hirose H, Kobayashi T, Okamura M, Kurauchi Y, Iwamura S, Uschijima T, Sawashima M. Recurrent laryngeal nerve palsy. *J Otolaryngol (Japan).* 1967;70:1–17.

Hiroto I, Hirano M, Tomita H. Electromyographic investigation of human vocal cord paralysis. *Ann Otol Rhinol Laryngol.* 1968;77:296–304.

Hiroto I, Hirano M, Toyozumi Y, Shin T. A new method of placement of a needle electrode in the intrinsic laryngeal muscles for electromyography. insertion through the skin. *Pract Otol (Kyoto).* 1962;55:499–504.

Hoffman HT, Brunberg JA, Winter P, Sullivan MJ, Kileny PR. Arytenoid subluxation: diagnosis and treatment. *Ann Otol Rhinol Laryngol.* 1991; 100(1): 1–9.

Holst M, Hertegard S, Persson A. Vocal dysfunction following crico-thyroidotomy; a prospective study. *Laryngoscope.* 1990;100(7): 749–755.

Holzer Se, Ludlow CL. The swallowing side effects of botulinum toxin type A injection in spasmodic dysphonia. *Laryngoscope.* 1996;106 (pt 1):86–92.

Howard JF, Sanders DB. Serial single-fiber EMG studies in myasthenic patients treated with corticosteroids and plasma exchange therapy. *Muscle Nerve.* 1983;4:254.

Hsiao TY, Solomon NP, Luschei ES, Titze IR. Modulation of fundamental frequency by laryngeal muscles during vibrato. *J Voice.* 1994;8(3): 224–229.

Inagi K, Ford CN, Rodriquez AA, Schultz E, Bless DM, Heisey DM. Efficacy of repeated botulinum toxin injections as a function of timing. *Ann Otol Rhinol Laryngol.* 1997;106(12):1012–1019.

Inagi K, Rodriquez M, Ford CN, Heisey DM. Transoral electromyographic recordings in botulinum toxin-injected rat larynges. *Ann Otol Rhinol Laryngol.* 1997;106(11):956–964.

Insalaco G, Kuna ST, Catania G, et al. Thyroarytenoid muscle activity in sleep apneas. *J Appl Physiol.* 1993;74(2):704–709.

Insalaco G, Kuna ST, Cibella F, Villeponteaux RD. Thyroarytenoid muscle activity during hypoxia, hypercapnia, and voluntary hyperventilation in humans. *J Appl Physiol.* 1990;69(1):268–273.

Insalaco G, Kuna ST, Costanza BM, Catania G, Cibella F, Bellia V. Thyroary-tenoid muscle activity during loaded and nonloaded breathing in adult humans. *J Appl Physiol.* 1991;70(6):2410–2416.

Isozaki E, Osanai R, Horiguchi S, Hayashida T, Hirose K, Tanabe H. Laryn-geal electromyography with separated surface electrodes in patients with multiple system atrophy presenting with vocal cord paralysis. *J Neurol.* 1994; 241(9):551–556.

Ito J, Kimura J, Shibasaki H. Palatopharyngolaryngeal myokymia resem-bling "palatal myoclonus" [letter]. *J Neurol Neurosurg Psychiatry.* 1993;56 (1):113–114.

Iwasaki H, Igarashi M, Namiki A, Omote K. Differential neuromuscular effects of vecuronium on the adductor and abductor laryngeal mus-cles and tibialis anterior muscle in dogs. *Br J Anaesth.* 1994;72(3): 321–323.

Jabre JF, Chirico-Post J, Weiner M. Stimulation SFEMG in myasthenia gravis. *Muscle Nerve.* 1989;12:38–42.

Jabre JF, Stalberg EV. Single-fiber EMG study of the flexor carpi radialis H reflex. *Muscle Nerve.* 1989;12:523–527.

Jaffe DM, Solomon NP, Robinson RA, Hoffman HT, Luschei ES. Comparison of concentric needle versus hooked-wire electrodes in the canine larynx. *Otolaryngol Head Neck Surg.* 1998;118(5):655–662.

Jankovic J, Schwartz K, Donovan DT. Botulinum toxin treatment of cranialcervical dystonia, spasmodic dysphonia, other focal dystonias and hemifacial spasm. *J Neurol Neurosurg, Psychiatry.* 1990;53(8): 633–639.

Johr M, Gerber H. Value of monitoring muscle relaxation. *Schweiz Med Wochenschr.* 1996;126(39):1649–1653.

Jonsson B, Reichmann S. Displacement and deformation of wire electrodes in electromyography. *Electromyography.* 1969;9:210–211.

Jurell KC. Surface EMG and fatigue. *Phys Med Rehabil Clin N Am.* 1998;9:933–947.

Kadefors R, Petersen I, Broman H. Spectral analysis of events in the electromyogram. In: Desmedt JE, ed. *New Developments in Electromyography and Clinical Neurophysiology.* Basel, Switzerland: Karger; 1973:628–637.

Kandel ER, Schwartz JH, Hessell TM. Ion channels. In: *Principles of Neuroscience.* 4th ed. New York, NY: McGraw-Hill; 2000:105–125.

Kandel ER, Schwartz JH, Hessell TM. Propagated signaling: the action potential. In: *Principles of Neuroscience.* 4th ed. New York, NY: McGraw-Hill; 2000: 150–175.

Kark AE, Kissen MW. Superior laryngeal nerve injury from thyroid surgery [letter to the editor]. *Head Neck.* 1995;17(6):542–543.

Kashima HK. Bilateral vocal fold motion impairment: pathophysiology and management by transverse cordotomy. *Ann Otol Rhinol Laryngol.* 1991;100(9 pt 1):717–721.

Kayamore R, Orii K. Schmidt syndrome due to idiopathic accessory nerve paralysis. *Electromyogr Clin Neurophysiol.* 1991;31(4):199–201.

Khan A, Pearlman RC, Bianchi DA, Hauck KW. Experience with two types of electromyography monitoring electrodes during thyroid surgery. *Am J Otolaryngol.* 1997;18(2):99–102.

Kimura J. *Electrodiagnosis in Diseases of Nerve and Muscles: Principles and Practice.* 2nd ed. Philadelphia, Pa: FA Davis Company; 1989.

King JC, Dumitru D, Nandedkar S. Concentric and single fiber electrode spatial recording characteristics. *Muscle Nerve.* 1990;20:1525–1533.

Knutsson E, Martensson A, Martensson B. The normal electromyogram in human vocal fold muscles. *Acta Otolaryngol (Stockh).* 1969;68: 526–536.

Kobayashi T, Niimi S, Kumada M, Kosaki H, Hirose H. Botulinum toxin treatment for spasmodic dysphonia. *Acta Oto-Laryngologica—Supplement* 1993;504:115–117.

Koch BM, Milmoe G, Grundfast KM. Vocal cord paralysis in children studied by monopolar electromyography. *Ped Neurol.* 1987;3(5):288-293.

Koda J, Ludlow CL. An evaluation of laryngeal muscle activation in patients with voice tremor. *Otolaryngol Head Neck Surg.* 1992;107(5): 684-696.

Kokesh J, Flint PW, Robinson LR, Cummings CW. Correlation between stroboscopy and electromyography in laryngeal paralysis. *Ann Otol Rhinol Laryngol.* 1993;102(11):852-857.

Konishi T, Nishitani H, Motomura S. Single fiber electromyography in chronic renal failure. *Muscle Nerve.* 1982;5:458-461.

Koufman JA, Postma GN, Cummins MM, Blalock FD. Vocal fold paresis. *Otolaryngol Head Neck Surg.* 2000;122(4)537-541.

Koufman JA, Postma GN, Whang CH, Rees CJ, et al. Diagnostic laryngeal electromyography: the Wake Forest experience 1995-1999. *Otolaryngol Head Neck Surg.* 2001;124(6):603-606.

Koufman JA, Walker FO, Joharji GM. The cricothyroid muscle does not influence vocal fold position in laryngeal paralysis. *Laryngoscope.* 1995;105(4 pt 1):368-372.

Krylov BS, Fel'berbaum RA, Ekimova GM. Characteristics of the motor innervation of the larynx. *Fiziol Zh SSSR.* 1983;69(4):481-488.

Kuna ST, Day RA, Insalaco G, Villeponteaux RD. Posterior cricoarytenoid activity in normal adults during involuntary and voluntary hyperventilation. *J Appl Physiol.* 1991;70(3):1377-1385.

Kuna ST, Insalaco G. Respiratory-related intrinsic laryngeal muscle activity in normal adults. *Prog Clin Biol Res.* 1990;345:117-124.

Kuna ST, Insalaco G, Villeponteaux RD. Arytenoideus muscle activity in normal adult humans during wakefulness and sleep. *J Appl Physiol.* 1991;70(4):1655-1664.

Kuna ST, Insalaco G, Villeponteaux RD, Vanoye CR, Smickley JS. Effect of hypercapnia and hypoxia on arytenoideus muscle activity in normal adult humans. *J Appl Physiol.* 1993;75(4):1781-1789.

Kuna ST, McCarthy MP, Smickley JS. Laryngeal response to passively induced hypocapnia during NREM sleep in normal adult humans. *J Appl Physiol.* 1993;75(3):1088-1096.

Kuna ST, Smickley JS, Vanoye CR, McMillan TH. Cricothyroid muscle activity during sleep in normal adult humans. *J Appl Physiol.* 1994;76(6): 2326-2332.

Kuna ST, Vanove CR. Laryngeal response during forced vital capacity maneuvers in normal adult humans. *Amer J Resp Crit Care Med.* 1994;150(3):729-734.

Lago P, Jone NB. Effect of motor unit firing time statistics on EMG spectra. *Med Biol Eng Comput.* 1977;15:648-655.

Laskawi R, Arold R, Damenz W. Diagnostic and prognostic significance of electromyography in laryngeal movement disorders. *Nervenarzt.* 1987;58(1):4-7.

Laskawi R, Arold R, Schroder M, Prange H. Practically relevant electrodiagnosis in facial and recurrent nerve pareses. a review. *Laryngol Rhinol Otol.* 1985;64(10):499-505.

Laukkanen AM, Lindholm P, Vilkman E. Phonation into a tube as a voice training method: acoustic and physiologic observations. *Folia Phoniatr Logop.* 1995;47(6):331-338.

Laukkanen AM, Lindholm P, Vilkman E, Haataja K, Alku P. A physiological and acoustic study on voiced bilabial fricative/beta:/as a vocal exercise. *J Voice.* 1996;10(1):67-77.

Lawry GV, Finerman ML, Hanafee WN, Mancuso AA, Fan PT, Bluestone R. Laryngeal involvement in rheumatoid arthritis. A clinical, laryngoscopic, and computerized tomographic study. *Arthritis Rheum.* 1984;27:873-882.

Lee RG, Ashby P, White DG, et al. Analysis of motor conduction velocity in the human median nerve by computer simulation of compound muscle action potentials. *Electroencephalogr Clin Neurophysiol.* 1975; 39:225-237.

LeFever RS, De Luca CJ. A procedure for decomposing the myoelectric signal into its constituent action potentials. I: Technique, theory and implementation. *IEEE Trans Biomed Eng.* 1982;29:149-157.

Levin KH, Luders HO. *Comprehensive Clinical Neurophysiology.* Philadelphia, Pa: W.B. Saunders; 2000.

Lewis JE, Olsen KD, Kurtin PJ, Kyle RA. Laryngeal amyloidosis: a clinicopathologic and immunohistochemical review. *Otolaryngol Head Neck Surg.* 1992;106:372-377.

Liguori R, Dhal K, Fuglsang-Frederiksen A. Turns-amplitude analysis of the electromyographic recruitment pattern disregarding force measurement I. method reference values in healthy subjects. *Muscle Nerve.* 1992;15:1314-1318.

Liguori R, Dahl K, Fuglsang-Frederiksen A, et al. Turns-amplitude analysis of the electromyographic interference pattern disregarding force management II. Findings in patients with neuromuscular disorders. *Muscle Nerve.* 1992;15:1319-1324.

Lindestad PA. Electromyographic and laryngoscopic studies of normal and disturbed voice function. *Studies in Logopedics and Phoniatrics No. 4.* Stockholm, Sweden: Huddinge University Hospital; 1994.

Lindestad PA, Fritzell B, Persson A. Evaluation of laryngeal muscle function by quantitative analysis of the EMG interference pattern. *Acta Oto-Laryngologica.* 1990;109(5-6):467-72.

Lindestad PA, Fritzell B, Persson A. Quantitative analysis of laryngeal EMG in normal subjects. *Acta Oto-Laryngologica.* 1991;111(6):1146-1152.

Lindestad PA, Fritzell B, Persson A. Influence of pitch and intensity on cricothyroid and thyroarytenoid activity in singers and nonsingers. In: Gauffin J, Hammarberg B, eds. *Vocal Fold Physiol—Acoustic, Perceptual and Physiological Aspects of Voice Mechanisms.* Singular Publishing Group: San Diego, Calif: 1991:175-182.

Lindestad PA, Hertegard S. Spindle-shaped glottal insufficiency with and without sulcus vocalis: a retrospective study. *Ann Otol Rhinol Laryngol.* 1994;103(7):547.

Lindestad PA, Hertegard S, Hammarberg B. An audioperceptual, videostroboscopic and electromyographic study of spindle-shaped glottal insufficiency with and without sulcus vocalis. *Phon Logoped Prog Rep.* 1994;9:21-32.

Lindestad PA, Persson A. Quantitative analysis of EMG interference pattern in patients with laryngeal paresis. *Acta Oto-Laryngologica.* 1994; 114(1):91-97.

Lindstrom LH, Magnusson RH. Interpretation of myoelectric power spectra: a model and its applications. *Proc IEEE.* 1977;65:653-662.

Lipton RJ, McCaffrey TV, Cahill DR. Sectional anatomy of the larynx: implications for the transcutaneous approach to endolaryngeal structures. *Ann Otol Rhinol Laryngol.* 1989;98(2):141-144.

Lipton RJ, McCafferty TV, Litchy WJ. Intraoperative electrophysiologic monitoring of laryngeal muscle during thyroid surgery. *Laryngoscope.* 1988;98 (12):1292-1296.

Lofqvist A, Yoshioka H. Laryngeal activity in Swedish obstruent clusters. *J Acout Soc Am.* 1980;68(3):792-801.

Lofqvist A, Yoshioka H. Interarticulator programming in obstruent production. *Phonetica.* 1981;38(1-3):21-34.

Lovelace RE, Blizter A, Ludlow C. Clinical laryngeal electromyography. In: Blitzer A, Brin MF, Sasaki CT, eds. *Neurologic Disorders of the Larynx.* New York, NY: Theime; 1992:66-82.

Ludlow C. Neurophysiological control of vocal fold adduction and abduction for phonation onset and offset during speech. In: Gauffin J, Hammarberg B, eds. *Vocal Fold Physiol—Acoustic, Perceptual and Physiological Aspects of Voice Mechanisms.* San Diego, Calif: Singular Publishing Group; 1991:197-205

Ludlow, CL. Treatment of speech and voice disorders with botulinum toxin (clinical conference). *JAMA.* 1990;264(20):2671-2675.

Ludlow CL, Naunton RF, Fujita M, Sedory SE. Spasmodic dysphonia: botulinum toxin injection after recurrent nerve surgery. *Otolaryngol Head Neck Surg.* 1990;102(2):122-131.

Ludlow CL, Naunton RF, Terada S, Anderson BJ. Successful treatment of selected cases of abductor spasmodic dysphonia using botulinum toxin injection. *Otolaryngol Head Neck Surg.* 1991;104(6):849–855.

Ludlow CL, Schultz GM, Yamashita T, Deleyiannis FW. Abnormalities in long latency responses to superior laryngeal nerve stimulation in adductor spasmodic dysphonia. *Ann Otol Rhinol Laryngol.* 1995; 104(12):928–935.

Ludlow CL, Van Pelt, Koda J. Characteristics of late responses to superior laryngeal nerve stimulation in humans. *Ann Otol Rhinol Laryngol.* 1992;101(2 pt 1):127–134.

Ludlow CL, Yeh J, Cohen LG, Van Pelt F, Rhew K, Hallett M. Limitations of electromyography and magnetic stimulation for assessing laryngeal muscle control. *Ann Otol Rhinol Laryngol.* 1994;103(1):16–27.

Manon-Espaillat R, Mandel S, Sataloff RT. Laryngeal electromyography. In: Sataloff RT. *Professional Voice: The Science and Art of Clinical Care.* 3rd ed. San Diego, Calif: Plural Publishing Inc; 2005;395–424.

Mao VH, Abaza M, Spiegel JR, Mandel S, Hawkshaw MJ, Heuer RJ, Sataloff RT. Laryngeal myasthenia gravis: report of 40 cases. *J Voice.* 2001; 15(1):122–130.

Marie JP, Dehesdin D, Ducastelle T, Senant J. Selective reinnervation of the abductor and adductor muscles of the canine larynx after recurrent nerve paralysis. *Ann Otol Rhinol Laryngol.* 1989;98(7 pt 1): 530–536.

Marion MH, Klap P, Perrin A, Cohen M. Stridor and focal laryngeal dystonia [see comment]. Comment in: *Lancet* 1992 Mar 28;339(8796):815. *Lancet* 1992 Feb 22;339(8791):457–458.

Martensson A, Skoglund CR. Contraction properties of intrinsic laryngeal muscles. *Acta Phys Scand.* 1964;60:318–336.

Massey JM, Sanders DB. Single-fiber EMG demonstrates reinnervation dynamics after nerve injury. *Neurology.* 1991;41:1150–1151.

Mazzantini M, Fattori B, Matteucci F, Gaeta P, Ursino F. Neuro-laryngeal involvement in Churg-Strauss syndrome. *Eur Arch Oto-Rhino-Laryngol.* 1998;255(6):302–306.

McComas AJ. Invited review. Motor unit estimation: methods, results and present status. *Muscle Nerve.* 1991;14:585–597.

McComas AJ. Motor-unit estimation: the beginning. *J Clin Neurophysiol.* 1995;12:560–564.

McComas AJ. Motorunit estimation: anxieties and achievements. *Muscle Nerve.* 1995;18:369–379.

McComas AJ, Fawcett PRW, Campbell MJ, et al. Electrophysiological estimation of the number of motor units within a human muscle. *J Neurol Neurosurg Psychiatry.* 1971;34:121–131.

McComas AJ, Sica RE, McNabb AR, Goldberg WM, Upton AR. Neuropathy in thyrotoxicosis. *N Engl J Med.* 1973;289:219-221.

McGill KC, Cummins KL, Dorfman LJ. Automatic decomposition of the clinical electromyogram. *IEEE Trans Biomed Eng.* 1985;32:470-477.

McGill KC, Dorfman LJ. Automatic decomposition electromyography (ADEMG): validation and normative data in brachial biceps. *Electroencephalogr Clin Neurophysiol.* 1985;61:453-461.

McGill K, Dorfman L. Automatic decomposition electromyography (ADEMG), methodologic and technical considerations. In: Desmedt JE, ed. *Computer Aided Electromyography and Expert Systems. Clinical Neurophysiology Updates.* Basel: Karger; 1989:91-101.

McGill KC, Lau K, Dorfman LJ. A comparison of terms analysis and motor unit analysis in electromyography. *Electroencephalogr Clinic Neurophysiol.* 1991;81:9-17.

McCulloch TM, Perlman AL, Palmer PM, Van Daele DJ. Laryngeal activity during swallow, phonation, and the Valsalva maneuver: an electromyographic analysis [published erratum appears in *Laryngoscope* 1997 Jan;107(1):146]. *Laryngoscope.* 1996;106(11):1651-1658.

McHenry MA, Kuna ST, Minton JR, Vanoye CR, Calhoun K. Differential activity of the pars recta and pars oblique in fundamental frequency control. *J Voice.* 1997;11(1):48-58.

Meikle D, Trachy RE, Cummings CW. Reinnervation of skeletal muscle: a comparison of nerve implantation with neuromuscular pedicle transfer in an animal model. *Ann Otol Rhinol Laryngol.* 1987;96(2 pt 1): 152-157.

Meleca RJ, Hogikyan ND, Bastian RW. A comparison of methods of botulinum toxin injection for abductory spasmodic dysphonia. *Otolaryngol Head Neck Surg.* 1997;117(5):487-492.

Mendell JR, Griggs RC. Muscular dystrophy. In: Wilson JD, Braunwald E, Isselbacher KJ, Petersdorf RG, Martin JB Fauci AS, Root RK, eds. *Harrison's Principles of Internal Medicine.* 12th ed. New York, NY: McGraw-Hill, Inc.; 1991:2112-2114.

Mihelin M, Trontelj JV, Stalberg E. Muscle fiber recovery functions studied in the double pulse stimulation. *Muscle Nerve.* 1991;14:739-747.

Miller Rh, Rosenfield DB. The role of electromyography in clinical laryngology. *Otolaryngol Head Neck Surg.* 1984;92:287-291.

Milner-Brown HS, Brown WF. New methods of estimating the number of motor units in a muscle. *J Neurol Neurosurg Psychiatry.* 1976;39: 258-265.

Milner-Brown HS, Stein RB, Yemm R. The orderly recruitment of human motor units during voluntary isometric contractions. *J Physiol (Lond).* 1973;230:359-370.

Min YB, Finnegan EM, Hoffman HT, Luschei ES, McCulloch TM. A preliminary study of the prognostic role of electromyography in laryngeal paralysis. *Otolaryngol Head Neck Surg.* 1994;111(6):770-775

Min YB, Luschei ES, Finnegan EM, McCullock TM, Hoffman HT. Portable telemetry system for electromyography. *Otolaryngol Head Neck Surg.* 1994;111(6):849-852.

Misiunas A, Niepomniszcze H, Ravera B, Faraj G, Faure E. Peripheral neuropathy in subclinical hypothyroidism. *Thryoid.* 1995;5:283-286.

Moorthy SS, Reddy RV, Dunfield JA, Radpour S, Dierdorf SF. The effect of muscle relaxants on cricothyroid muscle: a report of three cases. *Anesthes Analg.* 1996;82(3):657-660.

Mu LC, Yang SL. A new method of needle-electrode placement in the posterior cricoarytenoid muscle for electromyography. *Laryngoscope.* 1990;100(10 pt 1):1127-1131.

Nahm I, Shin T, Watanabe H, Maeyama T. Misdirected regeneration of injured recurrent laryngeal nerve in the cat. *Am J Otolaryngol.* 1993; 14(1):43-48.

Nandedkar SD, Barkhaus PE, Charles A. Multi-motor units action potential analysis. *Muscle Nerve.* 1995;18:1155-1166.

Nandedkar SD, Barkhaus PE, Sanders DB, et al. Analysis of the amplitude and area of concentric needle EMG motor unit action potentials. *Electroencephalogr Clin Neurophysiol.* 1988;69:561-567.

Nandedkar SD, Sanders DB. Measurement of the amplitude of the EMG envelope. *Muscle Nerve.* 1990;13:933-938.

Nandedkar SD, Sanders DB, Stalberg EV. Automatic analysis of the electromyographic interference pattern. Part I: Development of quantitative features. *Muscle Nerve.* 1985;8:431-439.

Nandedkar SD, Sanders DB, Stalberg EV. Automatic analysis of the electromyographic interference pattern. Part II: Findings in control subjects and in some neuromuscular disease. *Muscle Nerve.* 1985;8:491-500.

Nandedkar SD, Sanders DB, Stalberg EV. Selectivity of electromyographic recording techniques: a simulation study. *Med Biol Eng Comput.* 1985;23: 536-540.

Nandedkar SD, Sanders DB, Stalberg EV. Simulation and analysis of the electromyographic interference pattern in normal muscle. Part I: Turns and amplitude measurements. *Muscle Nerve.* 1986;9:423-430.

Nandedkar SD, Sanders DB, Stalberg EV. Simulation and analysis of the electromyographic interference pattern in normal muscle. Part II: Activity, upper centile amplitude and number of small segments. *Muscle Nerve.* 1986;9:486-490.

Nandedkar SD, Sanders DB, Stalberg EV, et al. Simulation of concentric needle EMG motor unit action potentials. *Muscle Nerve.* 1988;151-159.

Nandedkar SD, Sanders DB, Stalberg EV. On the shape of the normal turn-samplitude cloud. *Muscle Nerve.* 1991;14:8-13.

Nandedkar SD, Stalberg E. Simulation of macro EMG motor unit potentials. *Electroencephalogr Clin Neurophysiol.* 1983;56:52-62.

Nandedkar SD, Stalberg E, Kim YI, et al. Use of signal representation to identify abnormal motor unit potentials in macro EMG. *IEEE Trans Biomed Eng.* 1984;31:220-227.

Nash EA, Ludlow CL. Laryngeal muscle activity during speech breaks in adductor spasmodic dysphonia. *Laryngoscope.* 1996;106(4):484-489.

Neuschaefer-Rube C, Haase G, Angerstein W, Kremer B. Einseitige rekur-rensparese bei verdacht auf Lyme-borreliose [Unilateral recurrent nerve paralysis in suspected Lyme borreliosis]. *HNO.* 1995;43: 188-190.

Newsom-Davis J, Leys K, Vincent A, et al. Immunological evidence for the coexistence of the Lambert-Eaton myasthenic syndrome and myasthenia gravis in two patients. *J Neurol Neurosurg Psychiatry.* 1991;54: 452-453.

Nieman RF, Mountjoy JR, Allen EL. Myasthenia gravis focal to the larynx. report of a case. *Arch Otolaryngol.* 1975; 101:569-570.

Nirkko AB, Rosler KM, Hess CW. Sensitivity and specificity of needle electromyography: a prospective study comparing automated interference pattern analysis with single motor unit potential analysis. *Electroencephalogr Clin Neurophysiol.* 1995;97:1-10.

Palmer JB, Holloway AM, Tanaka E. Detecting lower motor neuron dysfunction of the pharynx and larynx with electromyography. *Arch Phys Med Rehabil.* 1991;72(3):214-218.

Palmer JB, Tippett DC, Wolf JS. Synchronous positive and negative myoclonus due to pontine hemorrhage. *Muscle Nerve.* 1991;14(2):124-132.

Parnes SM, Satya-Murti S. Predictive value of laryngeal electromyography in patients with vocal cord paralysis of neurogenic origin. *Laryngoscope.* 1985;95:1323-1326.

Paulsen FP, Jungmann K, Tillmann BN. The cricoarytenoid joint capsule and its relevance to endotracheal intubation. *Anesth Analg.* 2000;90: 180-185.

Paydarfar D, Gilbert RJ, Poppel CS, Nassab PF. Respiratory phase resetting and airflow changes induced by swallowing in humans. *J Physiol (Lond).* 1995;483(pt 1):273-288.

Philipsson L, Larsson P. The electromyographical signal as a measure of muscular force: a comparison of detection and quantification techniques. *Electromyogr Clin Neurophysiol.* 1988;28:141-150.

Pinelli P. Neurophysiology in the science of speech. *Cur Opin Neurol Neurosurg.* 1992;5(5):744-755.

Polisar IA. The crico-arytenoid joint. a diarthrodial articulation subject to rheumatoid arthritic involvement. *Laryngoscope.* 1959;69:1129–1164.

Polo A, Manganotti P, Zanette G, De Grandis D. Polyneuritis cranialis: clinical and electrophysiological findings. *J Neurol Neurosurg Psychiatry.* 1992;55(5):398–400.

Pototschnig C, Thumfart WF. Electromyographic evaluation of vocal cord disorders. *Acta Otorhinolaryngol Belg.* 1997;51(2):99–104.

Pototschnig CA, Schneider I, Eckel HE, Thumfart WF. Repeatedly successful closure of the larynx for the treatment of chronic aspiration with the use of botulinum toxin A. *Ann Otol Rhinol Laryngol.* 1996;105(7):521–524.

Pouderoux P, Logemann JA, Kahrilas PJ. Pharyngeal swallowing elicited by fluid infusion: role of volition and vallecular containment. *Am J Physiol.* 1996;270(2 pt 1):G347–G354.

Quiney RE. Laryngeal electromyography: a useful technique for the investigation of vocal cord palsy. *Clin Otolaryngol.* 1989;14(4)305–316.

Rabkin R. Paralysis of the larynx due to central nervous system syphilis. *Eye Ear Nose Throat Monthly.* 1963; 42:53.

Rea JL. Postcricoid surface laryngeal electrode. *Ear Nose Throat J.* 1992; 71(6):267–269.

Richardson MA. Developments in pediatric neurolaryngology. *Ann Otol Rhinol Laryngol.* 1997;96(1 pt 1):118–119.

Rieger A, Hass I, Gross M, Gramm HJ, Eyrich K. Intubation trauma of the larynx—a literature review with special reference to arytenoid cartilage dislocation. *Anasthesiol Intensivmen Notfallmed Schmerzther.* 1995;31(5):281–287.

Roark RM, Dowling EM, DeGroat RD, Watson BC, Schaefer SD. Timefrequency analyses of thyroarytenoid myoelectric activity in normal and spasmodic dysphonia subjects. *J Speech Hear Res.* 1995;38(2): 289–303.

Robinson LR, Hillel AD, Waugh PF. New laryngeal muscle weakness in postpolio syndrome. *Laryngoscope.* 1998;108(5):732–734.

Robinson JL, Mandel S, Sataloff RT. Objective voice measures in nonsinging patients with unilateral superior laryngeal nerve paresis. *J Voice.* 2005;19(4):665–667.

Rodriquez AA, Ford CN, Bless DM, Harmon RL. Electromyographic assessment of spasmodic dysphonia patient prior to botulinum toxin injection. *Electromyog Clin Neurophysiol.* 1994;34(7):403–407.

Rodriquez AA, Myers BR, Ford CN. Laryngeal electromyography in the diagnosis of laryngeal nerve injuries. *Arch Phys Med Rehab.* 1990; 71(8):587–590.

Ronager J, Christensen H, Fuglsang-Frederiksen A. Power spectrum analysis of the EMG pattern in normal and diseased muscles. *J Neurol Sci.* 1989;94:283–294.

Rontal E, Rontal M, Silverman B, Kileny PR. The clinical differentiation between vocal cord paralysis and vocal cord fixation using electromyography. *Laryngoscope.* 1993;103(2):133-137.

Rose A, Willison R. Quantitative electromyography using automatic analysis: studies in healthy subjects and patients with primary muscle disease. *J Neurol Neurosurg Psychiatry.* 1967;30:403-410.

Rossi G, Cortesina G. Morphological study of the laryngeal muscles in man: insertions and courses of the muscle fibers, motor end-plates and proprioceptors. *Acta Otolaryngol (Stockh).* 1965;59:575-592.

Roubeau B, Chevrie-Muller C, Lacau Saint Guily J. Electromyographic activity of strap and cricothyroid muscles in pitch change. *Acta Oto-Laryngologica.* 1997;117(3):456-464.

Rubin J, Sataloff RT, Kovovin G. *Diagnosis and Treatment of Voice Disorders.* San Diego Calif: Plural Publishing Inc; 2006.

Sadeh M, Kronenberg J. Gaton E. Histochemistry of human laryngeal muscles. *Cell Molec Biol.* 1981;27:643-648.

Sanders DB. The effect of firing rate on neuromuscular jitter in Lambert-Eaton myasthenic syndrome. *Muscle Nerve.* 1992;15:256-258.

Sanders DB, Howard JF. AAEM minimonograph #25: single-fiber electromyography in myasthenia gravis. *Muscle Nerve.* 1985;9:809-819.

Sanders DB, Massey EW, Buckley EG. Botulinum toxin for blepharospasm: single- fiber EMG studies. *Neurology.* 1986;36:545-547.

Sanders DB, Stalberg EV. AAEM minimonograph #25: single-fiber electromyograph. *Muscle Nerve.* 1996;19:1069-1083.

Sanders DB, Stalberg EV, Nandedkar SD. Analysis of the electromyographic interference pattern. *J Clin Neurophysiol.* 1996;13:385-400.

Sapir S, Larson KK. Supralaryngeal muscle activity during sustained vibrato in four sopranos: surface EMG findings. *J Voice.* 1993;7(3): 213-218.

Sataloff RT. *Professional Voice: The Science and Art of Clinical Care.* 3rd ed. San Diego, Calif: Plural Publishing Inc; 2005:1-798.

Sataloff RT. Clinical anatomy and physiology of the voice. In: Sataloff RT, *Professional Voice: The Science and Art of Clinical Care.* 3rd ed. San Diego, Calif: Plural Publishing Inc; 2005:143-178.

Sataloff RT, Bough ID, Spiegel JR. Arytenoid dislocation: diagnosis and treatment. *Laryngoscope.* 1994;104(10):1353-1361.

Sataloff RT, Emerich KA, Hoover CA. Endocrine dysfunction. In: Sataloff RT. *Professional Voice: The Science and Art of Clinical Care.* 3rd ed. San Diego, Calif: Plural Publishing Inc; 2005:537-550.

Sataloff RT, Feldman M, Darby KS, Carrol LM, Spiegel JR. Arytenoid dislocation. *J Voice.* 1987;1:368-377.

Sataloff RT, Mandel S., Gupta R. Neurological disorders affecting the voice in performance. *Professional Voice: The Science and Art of Clinical Care.* 3rd ed. San Diego, Calif: Plural Publishing Inc; 2005:847–890.

Satoh I. Evoked electromyographic test applied for recurrent laryngeal nerve paralysis. *Laryngoscope.* 1978; 88(12):2022–2032.

Schaefer SD, Roark RM, Watson BC, Kondraske GV, Freeman FJ, Butsch RW, Pohl J. Multichannel electromyographic observations in spasmodic dysphonia patients and normal control subjects. *Ann Otol Rhinol Laryngol.* 1992;101(1):67–75.

Scherer RS. Physiology of phonation: a review of basic mechanics. In: Ford CN, Bless DM, eds. *Phonosurgery.* New York, NY: Raven Press; 1991: 77–93.

Schiller HH, Stalberg EV. F responses studied with single fibre EMG in normal subjects and spastic patients. *J Neurol Neurosurg Psychiatry.* 1978;41:45–53.

Schiller HH, Stalberg E. Human botulism studied with single-fiber electromyography. *Arch Neurol.* 1978;35:346–349.

Schultz JL, Perlman AL, VanDaele DJ. Laryngeal movement, oropharyngeal pressure, and submental muscle contraction during swallowing. *Arch Phys Med Rehab.* 1994;75(2):183–188.

Schultz-Coulon HJ. Clinical course and therapy of congenital malformations of the larynx. *HNO.* 1984;32(4):135–148.

Schwartz MS, Moosa A, Dubowitz V. Correlation of single fibre EMG and muscle histochemistry using an open biopsy recording technique. *J Neurol Sci.* 1997;31:369–378.

Schwartz MS, Stalberg E. Myasthenia gravis with features of the myasthenic syndrome: an investigation with electrophysiologic methods including single-fibre electromyography. *Neurology.* 1975;25:80–84.

Schwartz MS, Stalberg E. Myasthenic syndrome studied with single fiber electromyography. *Arch Neurol.* 1975;32:815–817.

Schwartz MS, Stalberg E, Schiller HH, et al. The reinnervated motor unit in man. a single fibre EMG multielectrode investigation. *J Neurol Sci.* 1976;27:303–312.

Schweizer V, Woodson GE, Bertorini TE. Single fiber electromyography of the laryngeal muscles. *Muscle Nerve.* 1999;22(1):111–114.

Sercarz JA, Berke GS, Ming Y, Rothschiller J, Graves MC. Bilateral thyroarytenoid denervation: a new treatment for laryngeal hyperadduction disorders studied in the canine. *Otolaryngol Head Neck Surg.* 1992; 107(5): 657–668.

Shaw GY, Searl J, Hoover LA. Advances in the management of voice disorders. *Kansas Medicine.* 1994;95(12):274–277.

Shaw GY, Searl JP, Hoover LA. Diagnosis and treatment of unilateral cricothyroid muscle paralysis with a modified Isshiki type IV thyroplasty. *Otolaryngol Head Neck Surg.* 1995;113(6):679-688.

Shields RW. Single fiber electromyography in the differential diagnosis of myopathic limb girdle syndromes and chronic spinal muscular atrophy. *Muscle Nerve.* 1984;7:265-272.

Shields RW. Single fiber electromyography is a sensitive indicator of axonal degeneration in diabetes. *Neurology.* 1987;37:1394-1394.

Shenoy AM, Plinkert PK, Nanjundappa N, Premalata S, Arunodhay GR. Functional utility and oncologic safety of near-total laryngectomy with tracheopharyngeal speech shunt in a Third World oncologic center. *Eur Arch Otorhinolaryngol.* 1997;254(3):128-132.

Shindo ML, Herzon GD, Hanson DG, Cain DJ, Sahgal V. Effects of denervation on laryngeal muscles: a canine model. *Laryngoscope.* 1995; 102(6):663-669.

Shipp T, Doherty T, Morrissey P. Predicting vocal frequency from selected physiologic measures. *J Acoust Soc Am.* 1979;66:678-684.

Shipp T, Izdebski K, Reed C, Morrissy P. Intrinsic laryngeal muscle activity in a spastic dysphonia patient. *J Speech Hear Dis.* 1985;50(1):54-59.

Shuman CR, Weissman B. Recurrent laryngeal nerve involvement as a manifestation of diabetic neuropathy. *Diabetes.* 1968;17:302.

Sica RE, McComas AJ, Upton AR, et al. Motor unit estimation in small muscles of the hand. *J Neurol Neurosurg Psychiatry.* 1974;37:55-67.

Simpson DM, Kaufmann H, Sanders I, Wolfe DE. Laryngeal dystonia in multiple system atrophy [letter]. *Muscle Nerve.* 1992;15(10):1213-1215.

Simpson DM, Sternman D, Graves-Wright J, Sanders I. Vocal cord paralysis: clinical and electrophysiologic features. *Muscle Nerve.* 1993;16(9): 952-957.

Siribodhi C, Sundmaker W, Adkins JP, Bonner FJ. Electromyographic studies of laryngeal paralysis and regeneration of laryngeal motor nerves in dogs. *Laryngoscope.* 1963;73:148-163.

Sittel C, Stennert E, Thumfart WF, et al: Prognostic value of laryngeal electromyography in vocal fold paralysis. *Arch Otolaryngol Head Neck Surg.* 2000;127(2):155-160.

Smith A, Denny M, Shaffer LA, Kelly EM, Hirano, M. Activity of intrinsic laryngeal muscles in fluent and diffluent speech. *J Speech Hear Res.* 1996; 39(2):329-348.

Smith A, Luschei E, Denny M, Wood J, Hirano M, Badylak S. Spectral analyses of activity of laryngeal and orofacial muscles in stutterers. *J Neurol Neurosurg Psychiatry.* 1993;56(12):1303-1311.

Smith RJ, Neville MB, Bauman NM. Interarytenoid notch height relative to the vocal folds. pilot study. *Ann Otol Rhinol Laryngol.* 1994;103(10): 753-757.

Sonoo M, Stalberg E. The ability of MUP parameters to discriminate between normal and neurogenic MUPs in concentric EMG: analysis of the MUP "thickness" and the proposal of the "size index." *Electroencephalogr Clin Neurophysiol.* 1993;89:291-303.

Spiro J, Rendell JK, Gay T. Activation and coordination patterns of the suprahyoid muscles during swallowing. *Laryngoscope.* 1994;104(11 pt 1):1376-1382.

Stalberg E. Propagation velocity in human single muscle fibers in situ. *Acta Physiol Scan.* 70 1966;(suppl 287):1-112.

Stalberg E. Electrogenesis in human dystrophic muscle. In: Rowland LP, ed. *Pathogenesis of Human Muscular Dystrophies.* Amsterdam, Netherlands: Excerpta Medica; 1977:570-587.

Stalberg E. Macro EMG, a new recording technique. *J Neurol Neurosurg Psychiatry.* 1980;43:475-482.

Stalberg E. Electrophysical studies of reinnervation in ALS. In: Rowland LP, ed. *Human Motor Neuron Diseases.* New York, NY: Raven Press; 1982:47-59.

Stalberg E. Macroelectromyography in reinnervation. *Muscle Nerve.* 1982; 5:S135-S138.

Stalberg E. Macro EMG. *Muscle Nerve.* 1983;6:619-630.

Stalberg E. Single fiber EMG, macro EMG, and scanning EMG. new ways of looking at the motor unit. *Crit Rev Clin Neurobiol.* 1986;2:125-167.

Stalberg E. Use of single fiber EMG and macro EMG in study of reinnervation *Muscle Nerve.* 1990;13:804-813.

Stalberg E, Andreassen S, Falck B, et al. Quantitative analysis of individual motor unit potentials: a proposition for standardized terminology and criteria for measurement. *J Clin Neurophysiol.* 1986;3:313-348.

Stalberg E, Antoni L. Electrophysiological cross section of the motor unit. *J Neurol Neurosurg Psychiatry.* 1980;43:469-474.

Stalberg E, Antoni L. Microprocessors in the analysis of the motor unit and the neuromuscular transmission. In Yamazuchi N, Fijizawa K, eds. *Proceedings of the Conference on EEG and EMG Data Processing.* Amsterdam, Netherlands: Elsevier; 1981:295-313.

Stalberg E, Antoni L. Computer-aided EMG analysis. In: Desmedt JE, ed. *Progress in Clinical Neurophysiology.* Vol 10. Basel, Switzerland: Karger; 1983:186-234.

Stalberg E, Bischoff C, Falck B. Outliers, a way to detect abnormality in quantitative EMG. *Muscle Nerve.* 1994;17:392-399.

Stalberg E, Chu J, Bril V, Nandedkar S, Stalberg S, Ericsson M. Automatic analysis of the EMG interference pattern. *Electroenceophalogr Clin Neurophysiol.* 1983;56:672-681.

Stalberg E, Dioszeghy P. Scanning EMG in normal muscle and in neuromuscular disorders. *Electroencephalogr Clin Neuro Physiol.* 1991;81: 403-416.

Stalberg E, Ekstedt J. Single fibre EMG and microphysiology of the motor unit in normal and diseased human muscle. In: Desmedt JE, ed. *New Developments in Electromyography and Clinical Neurophysiology.* Vol 1. Basel, Switzerland: Karger; 1973:113-129.

Stalberg E, Ekstedt J, Broman A. The electromyographic jitter in normal human muscles. *Electroencephalogr Clin Neurophysiol.* 1971;31(5): 429-438.

Stalberg E, Ekstedt J, Broman A: Neuromuscular transmission in myasthenia gravis studied with single fibre electromyography. *J Neurol Neurosurg Psychiatry.* 1974;37:540-547.

Stalberg E, Falck B, Sonoo M, et al. Multi-MUP EMG analysis—a two year experience in daily clinical work. *Electroencephalogr Clin Neurophysiol.* 1995;97:145-154.

Stalberg E, Fawcett PR. Macro EMG changes in healthy subjects of different ages. *J Neurol Neurosurg Psychiatry.* 1992;45:870-878.

Stalberg E, Nandedkar SD, Sanders DB, et al. Quantitative motor unit potential analysis. *J Clin Neurophysiol.* 1996;13:401-422.

Stalberg E, Schwartz MS, Thiele B, et al. The normal motor unit in man. *J Neurol Sci.* 1976; 27:291-301.

Stalberg E, Schwartz MS, Trontelj JV. Singe fibre electromyography in various processes affecting the anterior horn cell. *J Neurol Sci.* 1975;24: 403-415.

Stalberg E, Sonoo M. Assessment of variability in the shape of the motor unit potential, the "jiggle," at consecutive discharges. *Muscle Nerve.* 1994;17:1135-1144.

Stalberg E, Thiele B. Transmission block in terminal nerve twigs: a single fibre electromyographic finding in man. *J Neurol Neurosurg Psychiatry.* 1972;35:52-59.

Stalberg E, Thiele B. Motor unit fibre density in the extensor digitorum communis muscle: single fibre electromyographic study in normal subjects of different ages. *J Neurol Neurosurg Psychiatry.* 1975;38: 874-880.

Stalberg E, Trontelj JV. Demonstration of axon reflexes in human motor nerve fibres. *J Neurol Neurosurg Psychiatry.* 1970;33: 571-579.

Stalberg E, Trontelj JV. *Single Fiber Electromyography in Healthy and Diseased Muscle.* 2nd ed. New York, NY: Raven Press; 1994.

Stalberg E, Trontelj JV, Mihelin M. Electrical microstimulation with single-fiber electromyography: a useful method to study the physiology of the motor unit. *J Neurophysiol.* 1992;9:105-119.

Stashuk D, DeLuca CJ. Update on the decomposition and analysis of EMG signals. In: Desmedt JE, ed. *Computer Aided Electromyography and Expert Systems. Clinical Neurophysiology Updates.* Vol 2. Basel: Karger; 1989:39-54.

Stashuk DW, Doherty TJ, Brown WF. EMG signal decomposition applied to motor unit estimates. *Muscle Nerve.* 1992;15:1191.

Stashuk DW, Doherty TJ, Kassam A, et al. Motor unit number estimates based on automated analysis of F responses. *Muscle Nerve.* 1994;17: 881-890.

Starmer CF, McIntosh HD, Whalen RE. Electrical hazards and cardiovascular function. *N Engl J Med.* 1973;289:219-221.

Stechison MT. Intraoperative monitoring of the vagus nerve during intracranial glossopharyngeal and upper vagal rhizotomy: technical note [letter; comment]. *Neurosurgery.* 1995;36(6):1238.

Sundberg J. *The Science of the Singing Voice.* DeKalb: Northern Illinois University Press; 1987:1-216.

Sussman HM, MCNeilage PG, Powers RK. Recruitment and discharge patterns of single motor units during speech production. *J Speech Hear Res.* 1977;20:613-630.

Tackmann W, Vogel P. Fibre density, amplitudes of macro-EMG motor unit potentials and conventional EMG recordings from the anterior tibial muscle in patients with amyotrophic lateral sclerosis. a study on 51 cases. *J Neurol.* 1988;235:149-154.

Tanaka S, Hirano M, Chijiwa K. Some aspects of vocal fold bowing. *Ann Otol Rhinol Laryngol.* 1994;103(5 pt 1):357-362.

Teitelbaum BJ, Wenig BL. Superior laryngeal nerve injury from thyroid surgery. *Head Neck Surg.* 1995;17(1):36-40.

Thiele B, Stalberg E. The bimodal jitter: a single fibre electromyographic findings. *J Neurol Neurosurg Psychiatry.* 1974;37:403-411.

Thiele B, Stalberg E. Single fibre EMG findings in polyneuropathies of different aetiology. *J Neuro Neurosurg Psychiatry.* 1975;38:881-887.

Thumfart W. Electromyography of the larynx. In: Samii M, Gannetta PJ, eds. *The Cranial Nerves.* Berlin, Germany: Springer-Verlag; 1981:597-606.

Thumfart W. Electrodiagnosis of caudal cranial nerve disorders in infants and small children. *Laryngol Rhinol Otol.* 1984;63(4):165-169.

Thumfart W, Gschwandtner R. Electroneurography of the laryngeal nerves in the awake patient using electromyography of the larynx under zoom-endoscopic-control (author's trans). *Laryngol Rhinol Otol (Stuttg).* 1980;59 (11):727-736.

Thumfart W, Steiner W, Jaumann MP. Electromyography of the cricoarytenoid muscle in the unsedated patient using the zoom-endoscope (author's trans). *HNO.* 1979;27(6):201–206.

Thumfart WF. Electromyography of the larynx and related techniques. *Acta Otorhinolaryngol Belg.* 1986;40(2):358–376.

Thumfart WF. From larynx to vocal ability. new electro-physiological data. *Acta Otolaryngol (Stockh).* 1998;05(5–6):425–431.

Thumfart WF, Pototschnig C, Zorowka P, Eckel HE. Electrophysiologic investigation of lower cranial nerve disease by means of magnetically stimulated neuromyography of the larynx. *Ann Otol Rhinol Laryngol.* 1992;101(8): 629–634.

Tiomny E, Khilkevic O, Korczyn AD, Kimmel R, Hallak A, Baron J, Blumen S, Asherov A, Gilat T. Esophageal smooth muscle dysfunction in oculopharyngeal muscular dystrophy. *Dig Dis Sci.* 1996;41(7): 1350–1354.

Titze IR, Luschei ES, Hirano M. The role of the thyroarytenoid muscles in the regulation of fundamental frequency. *J Voice.* 1989;3:213–224.

Topka H, Hallett M. Perioral reflexes in orofacial dyskinesia and spasmodic dysphonia. *Muscle Nerve.* 1992;15(9):1016–1022.

Torres CF, Moxley RT. Hypothyroid neuropathy and myopathy: clinical and electrodiagnostic in longitudinal findings. *J Neurol.* 1990;237: 271–274.

Trontelj JV. H-reflex of single motoneurones in man. *Nature.* 1968;220: 1043–1044.

Trontelj JV. A study of the H-reflex by single fibre EMG. *J Neurol Neurosurg Psychiatry.* 1972;36:951–959.

Trontelj JV. A study of the F response by single fibre electromyography. In: Desmedt JE, ed. *New Developments in Electromyography and Clinical Neurophysiology.* Vol 3. Basel, Switzerland: Karger; 1973:318–322.

Trontelj JV, Khuraibet A, Mihelin M. The jitter in stimulated orbicularis oculi muscle: technique and normal values. *J Neurol Neurosurg Psychiatry.* 1988;51:814–819.

Trontelj JV, Mihelin M, Fernandez JM, et al. Axonal stimulation for end-plate jitter studies. *J Neurol Neurosurg Psychiatry.* 1986;49:677–685.

Trontelj JV, Stalberg E. Bizarre repetitive discharges recorded with single fibre EMG. *J Neurol Neurosurg Psychiatry.* 1983;46:310–316.

Trontelj JV, Stalberg E. Single motor end plates in myasthenia gravis and LEMS at different firing rates. *Muscle Nerve.* 1991;14:226–232.

Trontelj JV, Stalberg E. Jitter measurements by axonal microstimulation. guidelines and technical notes. *Electroencephalogr Clin Neurophysiol.* 1992;85: 30–37.

Trontelj JV, Stalberg E, Mihelin M, et al. Jitter of the stimulated motor axon. *Muscle Nerve.* 1992;15:449–454.

Trontelj JV, Trontelj M. F-responses of human facial muscles. a single motorneurone study. *J Neurol Sci.* 1973;120:211–222.

Trontelj MA, Trontelj JV. Reflex arc of the first component of the human blink reflex: a single motorneurone study. *J Neurol Neurosurg Psychiatry.* 1978;41:538–574.

Truong DD, Rontal M, Rolnick M, Aronson AE, Mistura K. Double-blind controlled study of botulinum toxin in adductor spasmodic dysphonia. *Laryngoscope.* 1991;101:630–634.

Watson BC, McIntire D, Roark RM, Schaefer SD. Statistical analysis of electromyographic activity in spasmodic dysphonic and normal control subjects. *J Voice.* 1995;9(1):3–15.

Watson BC, Schaefer SD, Freeman FJ, Dembowski J, Kondraske G, Roark R. Laryngeal electromyographic activity in adductor and abductor spasmodic dysphonia. *J Speech Hear Res.* 1991;34(3):473–482.

Weddel G, Feinstein B, Pattle RE. The electrical activity of voluntary muscle in man under normal and pathological conditions. *Brain.* 1944; 67:178–257.

Weed, DT, Chongkolwatana C, Kawamura Y, et al. Reinnervation of the allograft larynx in the rat laryngeal transplant model. *Otolaryngol Head Neck Surg.* 1995;113(5):517–529.

Weed DT, Jewett BS, Rainey C, et al. Long-term follow-up of recurrent laryngeal nerve avulsion for the treatment of spastic dysphonia. *Ann Otol Rhinol Laryngol.* 1996;105(8):562–601.

Wellmeier W, Luba A, Schultz-Coulon HJ. The electromyography as an aid for the differential diagnosis of laryngeal movement disturbances (author's trans). *Laryngol Rhinol Otol (Stuttg).* 1979;58(4):353–360.

Wen W, Zhou S, Li Z. Experimental studies on the selective reinnervation of the abductor and adductor muscles of the larynx. *Chung Hua Erh Pi Yen Hou Ko Tsa Chih.* 1994;29(1):30–33.

Wheatley JR, Brancatisano A, Engel LA. Cricothyroid muscle responses to increased chemical drive in awake normal humans. *J Appl Physiol.* 1991;70(5):2233–2241.

Wheatley JR, Brancatisano A, Engel LA. Respiratory-related activity of cricothyroid muscle in awake normal humans. *J Appl Physiol.* 1991; 70(5): 2226–2232.

Willison R. Analysis of electrical activity in healthy and dystrophic muscles in man. *J Neurol Neurosurg Psychiatry.* 1964;27:386–394.

Willison RG. A method of measuring motor unit activity in human muscle. *J Physiol (Lond).* 1963;168:35–36P.

Willison RG. Analysis of electrical activity in healthy and dystrophic muscle in man. *J Neurol Neurosurg Psychiatry.* 1964;27:386–394.

Wolf SR. Electrode applicator for endolaryngeal electromyography of the larynx with local anesthesia. *Laryngorhinootologie.* 1995;74(7): 460–462.

Woo P, Arandia H. Intraoperative laryngeal electromyographic assessment of patients with immobile vocal fold. *Ann Otol Rhinol Laryngol.* 1992;101(10):799–806.

Woo P. Laryngeal electromyography is a cost-effective clinically useful tool in the evaluation of vocal fold function. *Arch Otolaryngol Head Neck Surg.* 1998;124(4):472–475.

Woodson GE. Clinical value of laryngeal EMG is dependent on experience of the clinician. *Arch Otolaryngol Head Neck Surg.* 1998;124(4):476.

Wozniak JA, Hutchison AA, Kosch, PC. Laryngeal and pump muscle activities during CO_2 breathing in neonates. *J Appl Physiol.* 1993;75(1): 416–423.

Yamanouchi H, Kasai H, Sakuragawa N, Kurokawa T. Palatal myoclonus in Krabbe disease. *Brain Dev.* 1991;13(5):355–358.

Yamashita T, Nash EA, Tanaka Y, Ludlow CL. Effects of stimulus intensity on laryngeal long latency responses in awake humans. *Otolaryngol Head Neck Surg.* 1997;117(5):521–529.

Yanagihara N, von Leden H. The cricothyroid muscle during phonation-electromyographic, aerodynamic and acoustic studies. *Ann Otol Rhinol Laryngol.* 1968;75:987–1006.

Yin SS, Qiu WW, Stucker FJ. Value of electromyography in differential diagnosis of laryngeal joint injuries after intubation. *Ann Otol Rhinol Laryngol.* 1996;105:446–451.

Yin S, Qiu WW, Stucker FJ, Batchelor BM. Critical evaluation of neurolaryngological disorders. *Ann Otol Rhinol Laryngol.* 2000;109(9):832–838.

Yokota J, Imai H, Seki K, Ninomiya C, Mizuno Y. Orthostatic tremor associated with voice tremor. *European Neurology.* 1992;32(6):354–358.

Ysunza A, Vazquez MC. Velopharyngeal sphincter physiology in deaf individuals. *Cleft Pal-Craniofac J.* 1993;30(2):141–143.

Zalewska E, Iiausmanowa-Petruseqicz I. Evaluation of MUAP shape irregularity—a new concept of quantification. *IEEE Trans Biomed Eng.* 1995;42:616–620.

Zheng H, Li Z, Zhou S. Ansa cervicalis to the adductor division of the recurrent laryngeal nerve anastomosis for unilateral vocal cord paralysis. *Chung Hua Erh Pi Yen Hou Ko Tsa Chih.* 1995;30(6):347–350.

Zheng H, Li Z, Zhou S, Cuan Y, Wen W. Update: laryngeal reinnervation for unilateral vocal cord paralysis with the ansa cervicalis. *Laryngoscope.* 1996;106 (12 pt 1):1522–1527.

INDEX